Springer
Berlin
Heidelberg
New York
Barcelona
Budapest
Hong Kong
London
Milan
Paris
Santa Clara
Singapore
Tokyo

Clay Smith

Gene Therapy
for HIV Infection

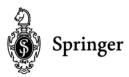 Springer

Clay Smith, M.D.
Director of Research
Bone Marrow Transplantation Program
Duke University Medical Center
Durham, North Carolina, U.S.A.

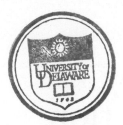

RC
607
,A26
G377
1998

ISBN: 3-540-64713-9 Springer-Verlag Berlin Heidelberg New York

Library of Congress Cataloging-in-Publication Data

Gene therapy for HIV infection [edited by] Clay Smith.
        p.   cm. -- (Biotechnology intelligence unit)
    Includes bibliographical references and index.
    ISBN 1-57059-540-2 (alk. paper)
    1. AIDS (Disease)--Gene therapy. 2. Immunogenetics. I. Smith, Clay, 1957- . II. Series.
    [DNLM: 1. HIV Infections--therapy. 2. Gene Therapy. WC 503.2 G326 1998]
RC607.A26G377 1998
616.97'92042--dc21
DNLM/DLC   98-23834
for Library of Congress   CIP

© Springer-Verlag Berlin Heidelberg and R.G. Landes Company, Georgetown, TX, U.S.A. 1998
Printed in Germany

The use of general descriptive names, registered names, trademarks, etc. in this publication does not imply, even in the absence of a specific statement, that such names are exempt from the relevant protective laws and regulations and therefore free for general use.

Product liability: The publisher cannot guarantee the accuracy of any information about dosage and application thereof contained in this book. In every individual case the user must check such information by consulting the relevant literature.

Typesetting: R.G. Landes Company, Georgetown, TX, U.S.A.

SPIN 10683868   31/3111 - 5 4 3 2 1 0 - Printed on acid-free paper

PREFACE

Since the early 1980s, the HIV epidemic has been raging within the United States and around the world.[1] Drug therapy for HIV infection has not been curative, prompting the search for alternative strategies to control HIV infection within infected persons. One potential alternative to drug therapy is a developing medical technology termed gene therapy.[2] Gene therapy involves introducing genetic elements into populations of cells in order to correct or prevent a pathologic process. A large number of gene therapy strategies have been developed in an attempt to inhibit HIV expression and spread. These strategies fall into two general categories, genetic modification of cells in order to elicit an immune response against HIV and genetic modification of the target cells of HIV infection in order to block HIV expression and reproduction.

In the first strategy, termed genetic immunotherapy by some, genetic material encoding HIV proteins is introduced into patient's cells in order to stimulate a cellular immune response above and beyond that stimulated by the viral infection itself.[3-5] Two general genetic immunotherapy strategies have been developed. Genes encoding HIV proteins have been directly injected into the dermis or muscle tissue of patients. These genes have been encoded in plasmids or viral DNA and have been injected either in the form of naked DNA or complexed with lipids. In the second approach, cells have been harvested from the patients, cultured ex vivo, genetically modified and then reinfused or injected back into the patients. In both strategies, the expressed HIV proteins are presumably taken up and processed by antigen presenting cells which then stimulate T-cell and B-cell responses through MHC restricted mechanisms. Currently clinical trials are underway to determine the safety and the efficacy of these approaches for treating HIV infection. Ultimately, these approaches may also be useful as a vaccine for individuals at high risk for HIV infection. This vaccination based approach to gene therapy for HIV infection has recently been reviewed and will be touched upon only briefly in this book.[6]

The second general HIV gene therapy strategy involves introduction of genetic elements into the target cells of HIV in order to directly block the spread and pathogenic actions of the virus.[7-11] For this strategy to be effective clinically, a variety of requirements must be satisfied. First, potent and safe genetic approaches to blocking HIV expression and replication must be developed. Second, the genetic elements which inhibit HIV must be efficiently introduced into the relevant target cells of HIV in such a way that they persist and are expressed at high levels for the lifespan of the cell. Since HIV infects a variety of hematopoietic cells including CD4+ T-lymphocytes, macrophages, dendritic cells, and microglial cells, genes must be delivered into each of these cells or their progenitors in order to fully block HIV. Since no effective methods have been developed yet for in vivo delivery of HIV inhibitory elements into these cell types or their progenitors, it is necessary to introduce these elements by collecting and manipulating the relevant cells ex vivo.[12-15] In order for the gene-modified cells to function after reinfusion into the patient, the ex vivo gene transfer process should not adversely affect the biology and immunologic activity of the genetically modified cells. Third, methods for safely and effectively transplanting the gene-modified cells must be developed, so that they persist and function within the patient at clinically relevant levels.[16] Fourth, given the expense and complexity of testing alternative gene therapy approaches in clinical trials, it is critical to develop efficient and informative preclinical models for testing the efficacy and safety of HIV gene therapy approaches.[17]

The purpose of this book is to address each of these issues in turn to provide a sense of the progress that has been made in this field and the challenges that remain in order for gene therapy strategies to become clinically effective for patients. In the first chapter, the biology of HIV will be reviewed in order to highlight specific aspects of the viral life cycle and the control of viral gene expression which could serve as targets for gene therapy strategies. In the second chapter, a summary of the variety of creative strategies that have been developed to block HIV gene expression and replication will be described. The third chapter describes trans-splicing ribozymes, a novel and exciting gene therapy approach which has been recently developed.

In the fourth chapter, several viral based gene delivery vectors, including murine retroviral vectors, lentiviral vectors, and adeno-associated viral vectors, will be described. These three systems are currently the only vectors capable of stably integrating into the cellular chromatin. Since the HIV gene therapy strategies described in this book all rely on expression of the inhibitory genetic elements for the lifespan of the cell and since many of the target cells for HIV infection are actively proliferating and have long lifespans, development of gene transfer vectors capable of stable integration in the host genome is essential.

The fifth and sixth chapters focus on issues related to introducing HIV genetic inhibitors into cells relevant to HIV infection, CD4 T-lymphocytes and hematopoietic stem cells. The purpose of introducing HIV genetic inhibitors into CD4+ T-lymphocytes would be to restore some degree of cellular immune function by infusing lymphocytes that could survive, proliferate and function, despite infection by HIV. The advantage of this approach is that T-cells are relatively easy to collect, culture ex vivo and infuse into the patient. The disadvantage is that even if an HIV genetic inhibition strategy were completely effective in the T-cells, a variety of other cell types would remain fully infectable by HIV, including macrophages, microglial cells, and dendritic cells. Since each of these cell types plays a critical role in maintaining immunity and also serves as a source for ongoing HIV infection, genetic protection of CD4+ T-cells alone would not restore or protect fully the immune system. In addition, the majority of gene-modified CD4+ T-cells probably only survive for days to months following reinfusion into the patient, necessitating multiple treatments. An attractive alternative to genetically modifying CD4+ T-lymphocytes would be to genetically modify pluripotent hematopoietic stem cells. These rare cells give rise to all other hematopoietic cells, including lymphocytes, macrophages, dendritic cells and microglial cells.[18] In addition, these cells have an enormous self renewal potential and are responsible for reconstituting the hematopoietic system for the lifespan of the recipient of a stem cell transplant. Despite these advantages, hematopoietic stem cells have been poorly characterized, and conditions for culturing and transducing them ex vivo have not been optimized. Chapter 6 discusses the biology of hematopoietic stem cells and strategies which may improve their characterization and genetic modification.

In addition to improving the potency of genetic HIV inhibition strategies and the delivery of these strategies into hematopoietic cells, it is essential to be able to compare alternative inhibitors and vectors in informative pre-clinical systems. This is particularly challenging with HIV, since the virus infects many cell types and much of the biology of HIV is based on complex interactions between the immune system and the virus which are difficult to recapitulate. Other complications are the complexity of the viral populations contributing to HIV infection and the absence of an analogous animal disease. The seventh chapter of this book will summarize the preclinical models which are currently available for evaluating the efficacy and safety of HIV gene therapy strategies.

The last chapter in this book will briefly summarize the field of hematopoietic stem cell transplantation, focusing on the clinical issues which are relevant to any HIV gene therapy approach involving transplantation of hematopoietic stem cells. There are a number of critical clinical considerations in achieving successful stem cell transplantation, including how best to treat the recipient so that the transplanted cells persist in clinically relevant numbers and how to minimize the toxicity of transplantation so that gene-modified stem cells could be successfully transplanted with acceptable morbidity and mortality.

In closing, I would like to comment briefly on the role that HIV gene therapy may play, given the significant improvements in understanding viral pathogenesis and in developing effective anti-viral drug development which have occurred over the past several years.[19,20] First, it has become clear that relatively quickly after initial infection, HIV becomes established in a variety of cell populations with differing biologies and lifespans.[21] In addition, HIV infects a much higher number of cells and is produced at much higher rates than originally appreciated.[22-24] Lastly, it appears that even though anti-viral therapies are becoming increasingly effective at blocking viral replication and spread, the immune system does not fully recover to its pre-infection competency.[25] Consequently, the later that anti-viral drug therapy is initiated in the course of HIV infection, the less likely it is that the immune system will recover.

Given these considerations, it now appears unlikely that introducing a population of gene-modified cells into a person with HIV infection would significantly reduce viral spread unless these cells comprised most or all of the hematopoietic system or had a selective advantage in vivo so that eventually they would replace most of the infected hematopoietic system. This goal does not appear achievable until pluripotent hematopoietic stem cells capable of reconstituting the entire hematopoietic system can be genetically modified at nearly 100% efficiency and then safely and effectively transplanted so that they replace the entire hematopoietic system of the HIV infected patient.[26] Consequently, gene therapy strategies may play a much more useful role in efforts aimed at immune reconstitution as opposed to efforts aimed at optimizing viral control. For example, gene therapy strategies could be incorporated in attempts to reconstitute the immune system of persons with HIV infection via adoptive transfer of T-lymphocytes or stem cells. In one such strategy, antigen specific ex vivo expanded T-cells could be infused into HIV infected persons with poor immunity to the pathogens which cause clinical problems in HIV infected persons. The most obvious candidates for this approach would be to generate and/or expand T-lymphocytes directed at cytomegalovirus (CMV) and Epstein Barr virus (EBV). These ex vivo expanded antigen specific T-cells would be infused into HIV infected persons with either indicators of limited immunity to these viruses or illnesses such as CMV retinitis or EBV related non-Hodgkin's lymphoma.[27-29] During the process of generating these antigen specific T-cells, genes conferring resistance to HIV could be introduced in order to prevent or retard destruction of the critical CD4+ helper T-cells by HIV following re-infusion of the ex vivo expanded T-cells into the patient. Clearly the success of such a strategy will depend on the potency of the HIV inhibitor as well as the extent to which the infused T-cells are destroyed by direct infection with HIV, as opposed to indirect mechanisms which cause T-cell destruction, including autoimmunity, superantigen driven T-cell proliferation and death, and T-cell apoptosis induced by HIV Env or Tat produced by neighboring infected cells.[30]

Clearly, the long term goal of HIV gene therapy approaches is to replace the need for continual and long term administration of multiple antiviral drugs. These drugs are difficult to take, have many side effects, and are costly. In addition, drug resistant HIV strains rapidly develop and even short interruptions in drug administration can lead to rapid disease relapses and progressive viral infection. This goal will ultimately be achieved when we understand how to genetically modify hematopoietic stem cells at high efficiency with potent HIV inhibitors so that they replace the endogenous, previously infected hematopoietic system. Exciting and rapidly advancing breakthroughs in improving genetic based inhibitors of HIV, gene delivery vectors, methods for manipulating and transplanting stem cells and in developing methods for directly modifying stem cells through in vivo gene delivery indicate that achieving this goal, while challenging, is only a matter of time.

References

1. Chin J. Present and future dimensions of the HIV/AIDS pandemic. 7th Interational Conference on AIDS, Florence 1991.
2. Mulligan R. The basic science of gene therapy. Science 1993; 260:926-932.
3. Winegar RA, Monforte JA, Suing KD, O'Loughlin KG, Rudd CJ, Macgregor JT. Determination of tissue distribution of an intramuscular plasmid vaccine using PCR and in situ DNA hybridization. Human Gene Therapy 1996; 7:2185-94.
4. Fuller DH, Murphey-Corb M, Clements J, Barnett S, Haynes JR. Induction of immunodeficiency virus-specific immune responses in rhesus monkeys following gene gun-mediated DNA vaccination. Journal of Medical Primatology 1996; 25:236-41.
5. Montgomery DL, Donnelly JJ, Shiver JW, Liu MA, Ulmer JB. Protein expression in vivo by injection of polynucleotides. Current Opinion in Biotechnology 1994; 5:505-10.
6. Piscitelli SC, Minor JR, Saville MW, Davey RT, Jr. Immune-based therapies for treatment of HIV infection. Annals of Pharmacotherapy 1996; 30:62-76.
7. Bridges SH, Sarver N. Gene therapy and immune restoration for HIV disease. Lancet 1995; 345:427-32.
8. Dropulic B, Jeang KT. Gene therapy for human immunodeficiency virus infection: genetic antiviral strategies and targets for intervention. Human Gene Therapy 1994; 5:927-39.
9. Gilboa E, Smith C. Gene therapy for infectious diseases: the AIDS model. Trends in Genetics 1994; 10:139-44.
10. Sarver N, Rossi J. Gene therapy: a bold direction for HIV-1 treatment. Aids Res Hum Retroviruses 1993; 9:483-7.
11. Yu M, Poeschla E, Wong-Staal F. Progress towards gene therapy for HIV infection. Gene Therapy 1994; 1:13-26.
12. Muench MO, Roncarolo MG, Namikawa R, Barcena A, Moore MA. Progress in the ex vivo expansion of hematopoietic progenitors. Leukemia and Lymphoma 1994; 16:1-11.

13. Moore MA. Review: Stratton Lecture 1990. Clinical implications of positive and negative hematopoietic stem cell regulators. Blood 1991; 78:1-19.

14. Haylock DN, Makino S, Dowse TL, Trimboli S, Niutta S, To LB, Juttner CA, Simmons PJ. Ex vivo hematopoietic progenitor cell expansion. Immunomethods 1994; 5:217-25.

15. Emerson SG. Ex vivo expansion of hematopoietic precursors, progenitors, and stem cells: the next generation of cellular therapeutics. Blood 1996; 87:3082-3088.

16. Reisner Y, Segall H. Hematopoietic stem cell transplantation for cancer therapy. Current Opinion in Immunology 1995; 7:687-93.

17. McCune JM. The SCID-hu mouse: a small animal model for the analysis of human hematolymphoid differentiation and function. Bone Marrow Transplant 1992; 1:74-6.

18. Krall WJ, Challita PM, Perlmutter LS, Skelton DC, Kohn DB. Cells expressing human glucocerebrosidase from a retroviral vector repopulate macrophages and central nervous system microglia after murine bone marrow transplantation. Blood 1994; 83:2737-48.

19. Terwilliger EF. Biology of HIV-1 and treatment strategies. Emergency Medicine Clinics of North America 1995; 13:27-42.

20. Schnittman SM, Fauci AS. Human immunodeficiency virus and acquired immunodeficiency syndrome: an update. Advances in Internal Medicine 1994; 39:305-55.

21. Embretson J, Zupancic M, Ribas JL, Burke A, Racz P, Tenner RK, Haase AT. Massive covert infection of helper T lymphocytes and macrophages by HIV during the incubation period of AIDS. Nature 1993; 362:359-62.

22. Piatak M, Jr., Saag MS, Yang LC, Clark SJ, Kappes JC, Luk KC, Hahn BH, Shaw GM, Lifson JD. High levels of HIV-1 in plasma during all stages of infection determined by competitive PCR. Science 1993; 259:1749-54.

23. Ho DD, Neumann AU, Perelson AS, Chen W, Leonard JM, Markowitz M. Rapid turnover of plasma virions and CD4 lymphocytes in HIV-1 infection. Nature 1995; 373:123-6.

24. Perelson AS, Neumann AU, Markowitz M, Leonard JM, Ho DD. HIV-1 dynamics in vivo: virion clearance rate, infected cell life-span, and viral generation time. Science 1996; 271:1582-6.

25. Collier AC, Coombs RW, Schoenfeld DA, Bassett RL, Timpone J, Baruch A, Jones M, Facey K, Whitacre C, McAuliffe VJ, Friedman HM, Merigan TC, Reichman RC, Hooper C, Corey L. Treatment of human immunodeficiency virus infection with saquinavir, zidovudine, and zalcitabine. AIDS Clinical Trials Group. New England Journal of Medicine 1996; 334:1011-7.

26. Smith C. Retroviral vector-mediated gene transfer into hematopoietic cells: prospects and issues. Journal of Hematotherapy 1992; 1:155-66.

27. Riddell SR, Walter BA, Gilbert MJ, Greenberg PD. Selective reconstitution of CD8+ cytotoxic T lymphocyte responses in immunodeficient bone marrow transplant recipients by the adoptive transfer of T cell clones. Bone Marrow Transplantation 1994; 14:S78-84.
28. Riddell SR, Greenberg PD. Therapeutic reconstitution of human viral immunity by adoptive transfer of cytotoxic T lymphocyte clones. Current Topics in Microbiology & Immunology 1994; 189:9-34.
29. Sing AP, Ambinder RF, Hong DJ, Jensen M, Batten W, Petersdorf E, Greenberg PD. Isolation of Epstein-Barr virus (EBV)-specific cytotoxic T lymphocytes that lyse Reed-Sternberg cells: implications for immune-mediated therapy of EBV+ Hodgkin's disease. Blood 1997; 89:1978-86.
30. Fauci A. The human immunodeficiency virus: infectivity and mechanisms of pathogenesis. Science 1988; 239:617-622.

CONTENTS

EDITOR

Clay Smith, M.D.
Director of Research
Bone Marrow Transplantation Program
Duke University Medical Center
Durham, North Carolina, U.S.A.
Chapter 8

CONTRIBUTORS

David Camerini, Ph.D.
Department of Microbiology and
Myles H. Thaler Center for AIDS
 and
Human Retrovirus Research
University of Virginia
Charlottesville, Virginia, U.S.A.
Chapter 7

Cristina Gasparetto, M.D.
Division of Oncology and
Transplantation Medicine
Duke University Medical Center
Durham, North Carolina, U.S.A.
Chapter 8

Tracy Gentry, M.T.(ASC P)
Division of Experimental Surgery
Duke University Medical Center
Durham, North Carolina, U.S.A.
Chapter 5

Magnús Gottfredsson, M.D.
Department of Medicine
Division of Infectious Diseases
Duke University Medical Center
Durham, North Carolin, U.S.A.
Chapters 1 and 2

Linda M. Kofeldt, M.D.
Department of Microbiology and
Myles H. Thaler Center for AIDS
 and Human Retrovirus Research
University of Virginia
Charlottesville, Virginia, U.S.A.
Chapter 7

Seong-Wook Lee, Ph.D.
Department of Molecular Biology
Dankook University
Seoul, Korea
Chapter 3

Kenneth L. Phillips
Division of Experimental Surgery
Duke University Medical Center
Durham, North Carolina, U.S.A.
Chapter 4

Robert Storms, Ph.D.
Division of Experimental Surgery
Duke University Medical Center
Durham, North Carolina, U.S.A.
Chapter 6

Bruce A. Sullenger, Ph.D.
Departments of Surgery and Genetics
Center for Genetic and Cellular
 Therapies
Duke University Medical Center
Durham, North Carolina, U.S.A.
Chapter 3

CHAPTER 1

Replicative Cycle of HIV

Magnús Gottfredsson

Introduction

Since the initial description of AIDS in 1981 and the subsequent discovery of HIV as the etiological agent in 1983, an enormous global effort has been put into research on this disorder and its prevention and treatment. In 1986 the first study was published demonstrating beneficial effects of drug treatment. However, until recently the benefits of drug treatment have been modest and short lived. Therefore, alternative therapeutic approaches have been proposed, such as gene therapy.

In the last 3 years we have witnessed an unprecedented progress in AIDS research, leading to improved understanding of viral dynamics and replication as well as significant advances in drug therapy, especially antiviral combinations of reverse transcriptase antagonists and protease inhibitors.[1,2] Despite these important advances several key questions regarding this disorder remain unanswered. For example, despite effective suppression of viral loads in HIV disease by using highly active antiretroviral therapy, complete normalization of immune function does not occur.[3] Furthermore, it is unknown whether lasting therapeutic effects can be achieved using combination drug therapy. Previous experience with antiretroviral agents suggests that emergence of resistance could become a problem unless viral replication is inhibited completely. In addition, toxicity with prolonged use of these agents could become prohibitive in the future, and combination therapies are extremely costly.[4-6]

Because of these problems there is still an impetus for research on alternative approaches in HIV infection, including gene therapy. Advances in drug therapy, as well as progress in our understanding

Gene Therapy for HIV Infection, edited by Clay Smith. © 1998 Springer-Verlag and R.G. Landes Company.

of the pathogenesis of HIV infection in the last 3 years, has led to the identification of new potential viral and cellular targets for gene therapy.[7] In addition, our understanding of the importance of immune function in HIV infection has improved. These advances are necessary foundations for improved gene therapeutic strategies and future progress in the field. In this chapter the replicative cycle of HIV will be reviewed. The emphasis will be on the viral components that have been successfully inhibited to suppress HIV replication.

HIV Replication and Genome Structure

HIV is a retrovirus belonging to the group lentiviridae.[8] It has recently become apparent that even during asymptomatic HIV infection the level of viral replication is much higher than previously thought. The lymph nodes are the main site for high-level virus production, producing over 1-10 billion virions every day and destroying a similar number of T cells in the process.[9,10] The genome of the HIV provirus is shown in Figure 1.1. It is bound by long terminal repeats (LTRs) at both the 5' and 3' ends of the genome. The LTRs consist of repeated segments which are termed U3, R and U5. The LTRs contain the promoter sequences and the transcript polyadenylation signal.[11] An overview of the HIV proteins and their function is given in Table 1.1.

Viral Binding and Entry

A schematic presentation of the replicative cycle of HIV is shown in Figure 1.2. The replicative cycle of HIV-1 starts by binding of the virus envelope glycoprotein (gp120) to CD4 on the cell surface.[12-14] Subsequently the viral envelope fuses with the cell membrane, a process which requires a cellular coreceptor. The chemokine receptors CCR-5 and CXCR-4 (formerly called Fusin) have been identified as the major coreceptors for HIV.[15-20] Macrophage-tropic strains of HIV, which constitute the vast majority of virus present in newly infected individuals, seem to use CCR-5, while T cell tropic strains, which generally appear late in the course of infection, use CXCR-4.[21-23]

Reverse Transcription

After fusion of the viral envelope with the cell membrane the viral core enters the cytoplasm, where viral RNA is immediately transcribed by reverse transcriptase (RT) into double-stranded DNA. The

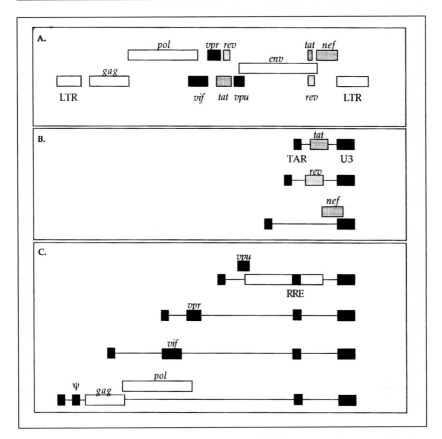

Fig. 1.1. A. Genome of the HIV provirus. It is bound by long terminal repeats (LTRs) at each 5' and 3' end of the genome. The LTRs consist of repeated segments which are termed U3, R and U5. The LTRs contain the promoter sequences and the transcript polyadenylation signal. B. Early mRNAs are mainly composed of doubly spliced transcripts encoding the regulatory proteins Tat, Rev and Nef. Each transcript begins with a trans-activating response (TAR) sequence at the 5' end and the U3 region of the LTR at the 3' end. C. Late gene expression includes singly spliced or unspliced mRNAs which encode the accessory proteins Vpu, Vif and Vpr. Each of the late mRNAs carries the Rev response element (RRE) sequence within the coding sequence of the env gene. The structural proteins (Gag-Pol) are encoded on a transcript which also carries the packaging sequence, ψ, located upstream from the *gag* gene. The Gag-Pol polyprotein is cleaved in the cytoplasm into structural proteins and viral enzymes by a viral protease.

RT enzyme has three enzymatic activities with essential functions for retrovirus replication: It is an RNA-dependent DNA polymerase (i.e., reverse transcriptase), but in addition it constitutes a DNA-dependent DNA polymerase activity (for synthesis of the second strand

Table 1.1. Proteins encoded by HIV-1

Gene	Virion proteins	Function
gag	Matrix protein, MA (p17)	Transport of preintegration compex in to nucleus
	Capsid protein, CA (p24)	Virus assembly
	Nucleocapsid, NC (p9)	RNA binding, virus assembly
pol	Protease, PR (p11)	Virus maturation
	Reverse transcriptase, RT (p66/p51)	Virus replication
	Integrase, IN (p32)	Virus replication
env	SU (gp 120)	Viral envelope, CD4 binding
	Transmembrane protein, TM (gp41)	Viral envelope, virus infectivity

	Accessory proteins	
vpr	Vpr	Translocation of preintegration complex to the nucleus (with MA) Cell cycle arrest in G2
nef	Nef	Downregulation of CD4 and MHC Class I
vif	Vif	Transport of incoming virus to the cell nucleus Packaging of nucleoprotein core into virions
vpu	Vpu	Enhancement of virion release Downregulation of CD4

	Regulatory proteins	
tat	Tat	Stimulation of viral transcription
rev	Rev	Regulator of late gene expression, transport of viral unspliced mRNA from nucleus to cytoplasm

Nuclear Import and Integration

After synthesis of the viral DNA, a nucleoprotein complex (or preintegration complex) containing the matrix protein, integrase and other viral proteins is translocated to the cell nucleus through connection with the cell nuclear import pathway.[24] The HIV accessory protein Vpr mediates transfer of the preintegration complex to the cell nucleus and probably enables the virus to infect nondividing cells.[24-26] After entry into the nucleus the viral DNA is integrated

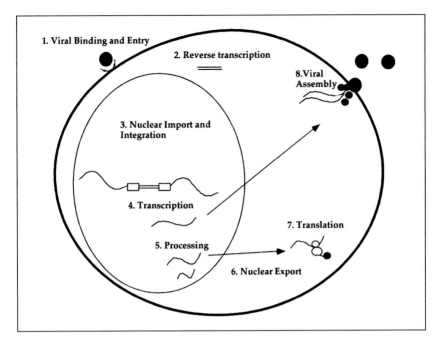

Fig. 1.2. Lifecycle of HIV.

cell nucleus and probably enables the virus to infect nondividing cells.[24-26] After entry into the nucleus the viral DNA is integrated into the host genome into regions of active transcription by the action of viral integrase.[27] In addition the integration process requires a newly identified host chromosomal protein.[28]

Transcription and Splicing

Following integration, the provirus is ready for LTR-regulated proviral gene expression, resulting in synthesis and proteolytic processing of structural proteins. Several viral regulatory proteins are important for viral replication (Table 1.1). The most important are Tat and Rev, but the accessory proteins Vpr, Nef, Vif and Vpu also have important roles.[24,29,30]

Tat protein interacts with its target sequence, termed the transactivation response element (TAR), a highly conserved 59 nucleotide RNA stem-loop structure that forms the 5' end of all HIV-1 transcripts.[30] Both Tat and TAR are essential for HIV replication in culture,[31-33] and binding by Tat to TAR RNA leads to an increase in HIV-1 transcription by greater than 100-fold.[34-36] Tat and TAR appear to form a complex which communicates with the transcription in the cell by binding to several components of the cellular transcription machinery.[37-41] Nuclear factor-κB (NF-κB) is an example of such a cellular transcription factor, which has been shown to act in concert with Tat to stimulate HIV RNA synthesis.[42] It increases the transcription of genes linked to the HIV LTR by enhanced transcription elongation and transcription initiation.[30] Early on in the viral replicative cycle, the HIV RNA transcripts are spliced multiple times by the cellular splicing machinery. The Rev and Nef proteins are produced from these multiply spliced transcripts and subsequently start to accumulate.

Rev is a 116 amino-acid protein which is localized in the nuclei and nucleoli of expressing cells and binds to a stem loop in the Rev Response Element (RRE), a 210 nucleotide HIV RNA sequence.[30,43] It has been shown that the Rev peptide has an alpha-helical conformation and binds in the major groove of the RRE near a purine-rich internal loop.[44] Binding of Rev to the RRE leads to a progressive shift in viral mRNA production from multiply spliced (encoding Tat, Rev and Nef) to unspliced transcripts which function as the virion RNA and the mRNA for the Gag-Pol polyprotein late in infection.[30]

The unspliced viral mRNA is transported from the nucleus to the cytoplasm, where viral structural proteins are subsequently synthesized (Fig. 1.3).[30,45] The Rev protein is required for this export of singly spliced and unspliced viral RNA.[30,45] A nuclear export signal has been identified in the Rev protein[46,47] which presumably recognizes and binds to exportin 1, a cellular nuclear export factor.[48-50] Presumably, exportin 1 shuttles the Rev-RNA complex from the nucleus to the cytoplasm where translation occurs (Fig. 1.3). However, other cellular factors are probably involved in Rev-dependent RNA transport, such as the Rev/Rex activation domain-binding (RAB) protein[51] and Rev-interacting protein (Rip1p), a small nucleoporin-like protein.[52,53]

The Nef protein has gained attention as a potential drug target, since it is important for maintenance of high viral loads and for the development of AIDS.[54] Clinical observations on patients infected with HIV isolates that contain deletions in their *nef* gene show that viral loads are remarkably low and the subjects remain asymptomatic for extended periods of time.[55] HIV infection leads to downregulation of surface expression of MHC-I and CD4 by endocytosis of molecules from the cell surface.[56-59] It has recently been shown

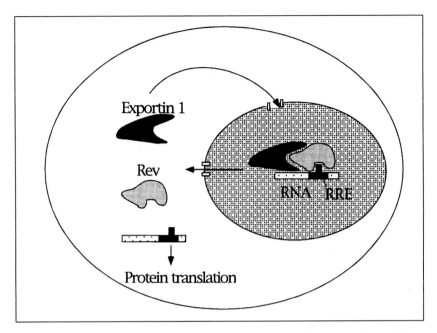

Fig. 1.3. Rev-mediated export of HIV RNA. The unspliced viral mRNA is shuttled from the nucleus to the cytoplasm by exportin 1. The complex is broken down in the cytoplasm where viral proteins are synthesized.

that these effects are mediated by the Nef protein.[59,60] The stimulation of endocytosis by Nef could therefore represent a viral mechanism for evading the immune response, because downregulation of MHC-I molecules makes HIV-infected cells less susceptible to lysis by CTLs.[56,57] In addition, human-PBL-SCID mice infected with mutants lacking the *nef* gene exhibit delayed CD4+ T cell depletion.[61]

Translation

Once in the cytoplasm the unspliced viral mRNA is translated into a Gag-Pol polyprotein by ribosomal frame shifting. The Gag-Pol polyprotein is cleaved by the viral protease into the mature virion structural proteins (matrix, capsid, and nucleocapsid) as well as the virion enzymes (protease, reverse transcriptase and integrase).[62] The viral envelope is synthesized as the gp160 precursor polyprotein, which is subsequently cleaved by cellular proteases into the external surface protein gp120 and a transmembrane protein gp41.

Viral Assembly

Assembly of the virions can then take place. The Vif accessory protein binds to the Pr55^{Gag} precursors[63] and binds to the host cell membrane. The Gag proteins thus accumulate at the inner surface of the cellular membrane and in turn bind retroviral RNA. This binding involves an interaction between RNA packaging signal sequences (ψ) and the zinc binding domains of the nucleocapsid protein.[27,64] The efficient packaging of retroviral RNA into virions requires an intact ψ packaging sequence.[65,66] The virus assembly seems to be regulated in part by the accessory protein Vpu (maturation protein).[67]Since the viral gp120 is able to bind to CD4 intracellularly, this interaction traps the protein and reduces its levels. The Vpu protein reduces the formation of intracellular gp120-CD4 complexes by degradation of the CD4 molecule. Subsequently, new virions are released from the surface of the host cell by budding and a new cycle of infection can start.

Acknowledgments

I thank Dr. Paul R. Bohjanen for helpful comments on the manuscript. MG is supported in part by a NATO science fellowship.

References

1. Cavert W, Notermans DW, Staskus K et al. Kinetics of response in lymphod tissues to antiretroviral therapy of HIV-1 infection. Science 1997; 276:960-964.
2. Gulick RM, Mellors JW, Havlir D et al. Treatment with indinavir, zidovudine, and lamivudine in adults with human immunodeficiency virus infection and prior antiretroviral therapy. N Engl J Med 1997; 337:734-739.
3. Autran B, Carcekain G, Li TS et al. Positive effects of combined antiretroviral therapy on CD4+ T cell homeostasis and function in advanced HIV disease. Science 1997; 277:112-116.
4. Schmit J-C, Ruiz L, Clotet B et al. Resistance-related mutations in the HIV-1 protease gene of patients treated for 1 year with the protease inhibitor ritonavir (ABT-538). AIDS 1996; 10:995-999.
5. Condra JH, Schleif WA, Blahy OM et al. In vivo emergence of HIV-1 variants resistant to multiple protease inhibitors. Nature 1995; 374:569-571.
6. Markowitz M, Mo H, Kempf DJ et al. Selection and analysis of human immunodeficiency virus type 1 variants with increased resistance to ABT-538, a novel protease inhibitor. J Virol 1995; 69:701-706.
7. Gottfredsson M, Bohjanen PR. Human immunodeficiency virus type 1 as a target for gene therapy. Front Biosci 1997; 2:D619-634.

8. Gallo RC. Human retroviruses in the second decade: a personal perspective. Nature Med 1995; 1:753-759.
9. Ho DD, Neumann AU, Perelson AS et al. Rapid turnover of plasma virions and CD4 lymphocytes in HIV-1 infection. Nature 1995; 373:123-126.
10. Wei X, Ghosh SK, Taylor ME et al. Viral dynamics in human immunodeficiency virus type 1 infection. Nature 1995; 373:117-122.
11. Buchschacher GL Jr. Molecular targets of gene transfer therapy for HIV infection. JAMA 1993; 269:2880-2886.
12. Maddon PJ, Dalgleish AG, McDougal JS et al. The T4 gene encodes the AIDS virus receptor and is expressed in the immune system and the brain. Cell 1986; 47:333-348.
13. Dalgleish AG, Beverley PCL, Clapham PR et al. The CD4 (T4) antigen is an essential component of the receptor for the AIDS retrovirus. Nature 1984; 312:763-767.
14. Klatzman D, Champagne E, Chamaret S et al. T lymphocyte T4 molecule behaves as the receptor for human retrovirus LAV. Nature 1984; 312:767-768.
15. Alkhatib G, Combardiere C, Broder CC et al. CC CKR5: A RANTES, MIP-1α, MIP-1β receptor as a fusion cofactor for macrophage-tropic HIV-1. Science 1996; 272:1955-1958.
16. Choe H, Farzan M, Sun Y et al. The β-Chemokine receptors CCR3 and CCR5 facilitate infection by primary HIV-1 isolates. Cell 1996; 85:1135-1148.
17. Deng H, Liu R, Ellmeier W et al. Identification of a major coreceptor for primary isolates of HIV-1. Nature 1996; 381:661-666.
18. Doranz BJ, Rucker J, Yi Y et al. A dual-tropic primary HIV-1 isolate that uses Fusin and the β-Chemokine receptors CKR-5, CKR-3, and CKR-2b as Fusion cofactors. Cell 1996; 85:1149-1158.
19. Dragic T, Litwin V, Allaway GP et al. HIV-1 entry into CD4+ cells is mediated by the chemokine receptor CC-CKR-5. Nature 1996; 381:667-673.
20. Feng Y, Broder CC, Kennedy PE et al. HIV-1 entry cofactor: Functional cDNA cloning of a seven-transmembrane, G protein-coupled receptor. Science 1996; 272:872-877.
21. Zhu T, Mo H, Wang N et al. Genotypic and phenotypic characterization of HIV-1 in patients with primary infection. Science 1993; 261:1179-1181.
22. Schuitemaker H, Koot M, Koostra NA et al. Biological phenotype of human immunodeficiency virus type 1 clones at different stages of infection: progression of disease is associated with a shift from monocytotropic to T cell tropic virus populations. J Virol 1992; 66:1354-1360.
23. Connor RI, Ho DD. Human immunodeficiency virus type 1 variants with increased replicative capacity develop during the asymptomatic stage before disease progression. J Virol 1994; 68:4400-4408.

24. Trono D. HIV accessory proteins: leading roles for the supporting cast. Cell 1995; 82:189-192.

25. Heinzinger NK, Bukrinsky MI, Haggerty SA et al. The Vpr protein of human immunodeficiency virus type 1 influences nuclear localization of viral nucleic acids in nondividing host cells. Proc Natl Acad Sci USA 1994; 91:7311-7315.

26. Miller RH, Turk SR, Black RJ et al. Conference summary: novel HIV therapies—from discovery to clinical proof of concept. AIDS Res Hum Retroviruses 1996; 12:859-865.

27. Karn J. An introduction to the growth cycle of human immunodeficiency virus. In: Karn J, ed. HIV. Biochemistry, molecular biology, and drug discovery. Vol. 2. Oxford: Oxford University Press, 1995:3-14.

28. Farnet CM, Bushman FD. HIV-1 cDNA integration: requirement of HMG I(Y) protein for function of preintegration complexes in vitro. Cell 1997; 88:483-492.

29. Cullen BR. The HIV-1 Tat protein: an RNA sequence-specific processivity factor? Cell 1990; 63:655-657.

30. Cullen BR. Mechanism of action of regulatory proteins encoded by complex retroviruses. Microbiol Rev 1992; 56:375-394.

31. Dayton AI, Sodorski JG, Rosen CA et al. The trans-activator gene of the human T cell lymphotropic virus type III is required for replication. Cell 1986; 44:941-947.

32. Fisher AG, Feinberg MB, Josephs SF et al. The trans-activator gene of HTLV-III is essential for virus replication. Nature 1986; 320:367-371.

33. Rosen CA, Sodorski JG, Haseltine WA. The location of cis-acting regulatory sequences in the human T cell lymphotropic virus type III (HTLV-III/LAV) long terminal repeat. Cell 1985; 41:813-823.

34. Feng S, Holland EC. HIV-1 tat trans-activation requires the loop sequence within tar. Nature 1988; 334:165-167.

35. Cullen BR. Trans-activation of human immunodeficiency virus occurs via a bimodal mechanism. Cell 1986; 46:973-982.

36. Arya SK, Guo C, Josephs SF et al. Trans-activator gene of human T-lymphotropic virus type III (HTLV-III). Science 1985; 229:69-73.

37. Garcia-Martinez LF, Ivanov D et al. Association of Tat with purified HIV-1 and HIV-1 transcription preintegration complexes. J Biol Chem 1997; 272:6851-6958.

38. Mavankal G, Ignatius Ou SH, Oliver H et al. Human immunodeficiency virus type 1 and 2 Tat proteins specifically interact with RNA polymerase II. Proc Natl Acad Sci USA 1996; 93:2089-2094.

39. Parada CA, Roeder RG. Enhanced processivity of RNA polymerase II triggered by Tat-induced phosphorylation of its carboxy-terminal domain. Nature 1996; 384:375-378.

40. Jeang KT, Chun R, Lin NH et al. In vitro and in vivo binding of human immunodeficiency virus type 1 Tat protein and Sp1 transcription factor. J Virol 1993; 67:6224-6233.

41. Kashanchi F, Piras G, Radonovich MF et al. Direct interaction of human TFIID with the HIV-1 transactivator tat. Nature 1994; 367:295-299.
42. Liu J, Perkins ND, Schmid RM et al. Specific NF-κB subunits act in concert with tat to stimulate human immunodeficiency virus type 1 infection. J Virol 1992; 66:3883-3887.
43. Daly TJ, Cook KS, Gray GS et al. Specific binding of HIV-1 recombinant Rev protein to the Rev-response element in vitro. Nature 1989; 342:816-819.
44. Battiste JL, Mao H, Rao S et al. Alpha helix-RNA major groove recognition in an HIV-1 Rev peptide-RRE RNA complex. Science 1996; 273:1547-1551.
45. Malim MH, Hauber J, Le S-Y et al. The HIV-1 *rev* trans-activator acts through a structured target sequence to activate nuclear export of unspliced viral mRNA. Nature 1989; 338:254-257.
46. Wen W, Meinkoth JL, Tsien RY et al. Identification of a signal for rapid export of proteins from nucleus. Cell 1995; 82:463-473.
47. Fisher U, Huber J, Boelens WC et al. The HIV-1 Rev activation domain is a nuclear export signal that accesses an export pathway used by specific cellular RNAs. Cell 1995; 82:475-483.
48. Ullman KS, Powers MA, Forbes DJ. Nuclear export receptors: From importin to exportin. Cell 1997; 90:967-970.
49. Stade K, Ford CS, Guthrie C et al. Exportin 1 (Crm1p) is an essential nuclear export factor. Cell 1997; 90:1041-1050.
50. Fornerod M, Ohno M, Yoshida M et al. CRM1 is an export receptor for leucine-rich nuclear export signals. Cell 1997; 90:1051-1060.
51. Bogerd HP, Fridell RA, Madore S et al. Identification of a novel cellular cofactor for the rev/rex class of retroviral regulatory proteins. Cell 1995; 82:485-494.
52. Stutz F, Neville M, Rosbash M. Identification of a novel nuclear pore-associated protein as a functional target of the HIV-1 rev protein in yeast. Cell 1995; 82:495-506.
53. Fritz CC, Zapp ML, Green MR. A human nucleoporin-like protein that specifically interacts with HIV Rev. Nature 1995; 376:530-533.
54. Kestler HW III, Ringler DJ, Mori K et al. Importance of the *nef* gene for maintenance of high virus loads and for development of AIDS. Cell 1991; 65:651-662.
55. Deacon NJ, Tsykin A, Solomon A et al. Genomic structure of an attenuated quasi species of HIV-1 from a blood transfusion donor and recipients. Science 1995; 270:988-991.
56. Kerkau T, Schmitt-Landgraf R et al. Downregulation of HLA class I antigens in HIV-1-infected cells. AIDS Res Hum Retroviruses 1989; 5:613-620.
57. Scheppler JA, Nicholson JKA, Swan DC et al. Down-modulation of MHC-I in a CD4+ T cell line, CEM-E5, after HIV-1 infection. J Immunol 1989; 143:2858-2866.

58. Garcia JV, Miller AD. Serine phosphorylation-independent down-regulation of cell-surface CD4 by *nef.* Nature 1991; 350:508-511.
59. Aiken C, Konner J, Landau NR et al. Nef induces CD4 endocytosis: requirement for a critical dileucine motif in the membrane-proximal CD4 cytoplasmic domain. Cell 1994; 76:853-864.
60. Schwartz O, Maréchal V, Le Gall S et al. Endocytosis of major histocompatibility complex class I molecules is induced by the HIV-1 nef protein. Nature Med 1996; 2:338-342.
61. Gulizia RJ, Collman RG, Levy JA et al. Deletion of *nef* slows but does not prevent CD4-positive T cell depletion in human immunodeficiency virus type 1-infected human-PBL-SCID mice. J Virol 1997; 71:4161-4164.
62. Debouck C, Tomaszek TA Jr, Ivanoff LA et al. HIV protease. In: Karn J, ed. HIV. Biochemistry, molecular biology and drug discovery. Vol. 2. Oxford: Oxford University Press, 1995:73-88.
63. Bouyac M, Courcoul M, Bertoia G et al. Human immunodeficiency virus type 1 vif protein binds to the pr55gag precursor. J Virol 1997; 71:9358-9365.
64. Rice WG, Supko JG, Malspeis L et al. Inhibitors of HIV nucleoprotein Zinc fingers as candidates for the treatment of AIDS. Science 1995; 270:1194-1197.
65. Lever A, Gottlinger H, Haseltine W et al. Identification of a sequence required for efficient packaging of human immunodeficiency virus type 1 RNA into virions. J Virol 1989; 63:4085-4087.
66. Mann R, Baltimore D. Varying the position of a retrovirus packaging sequence results in the encapsidation of both unspliced and spliced RNAs. J Virol 1985; 54:401-407.
67. Chen BK, Gandhi RT, Baltimore D. CD4 down-modulation during infection of human T cells with human immunodeficiency virus type 1 involves independent activities of *vpu, env* and *nef.* J Virol 1996; 70:6044-6053.

CHAPTER 2

Gene Therapy Strategies for Inhibition of HIV

Magnús Gottfredsson

Introduction

Most of the HIV proteins and virtually every stage in the HIV life cycle can be viewed as a potential site for inhibition. Several of the HIV proteins have been successfully inhibited in vitro and in T cell lines. However, challenging transduced primary T cells and macrophages with diverse strains of HIV is a more realistic system to test and compare the effectiveness of different gene therapy approaches. With several clinical trials planned or underway, the field of gene therapy research for HIV disease is very active, representing 18% of patients undergoing clinical gene therapy trials.[1] These advances parallel the remarkable progress in stem cell biology in the past 2-3 years.[2,3] In the future, once an ideal combination of anti-HIV genes has been identified, stem cells could be made resistant by one-time delivery of potent combinations of antiviral genes, thereby reconstituting an immune system durably protected from rampant viral multiplication. This chapter reviews different gene therapy approaches that have been taken to inhibit HIV replication, using either viral components or cellular proteins as targets.

Inhibition Strategies

As the terminology may be new to some readers, a brief explanation of the terms is in order. Specific examples of their applications will be subsequently reviewed in each section of this chapter:

Gene Therapy for HIV Infection, edited by Clay Smith. © 1998 Springer-Verlag and R.G. Landes Company.

1. Intracellular immunization. This term has been reserved for strategies where intracellular antibodies or antibody fragments ("intrabodies") are used to neutralize a specific target, such as the enzyme reverse transcriptase or the gp120 protein.

2. Transdominant negative mutant proteins. The viral proteins Tat and Rev contain domains which have been characterized with respect to structure and function. Viral replication has been successfully inhibited by intracellularly expressing mutant proteins lacking the transactivation domains.

3. RNA decoys. As outlined in Chapter 1, the Tat and Rev proteins bind to highly conserved areas in the HIV transcripts, TAR and RRE, respectively. The term RNA decoys has been reserved for RNA molecules which mimic crucial areas in the authentic TAR and RRE sequences. The decoys lead to competitive inhibition in viral replication by binding the Tat and Rev regulatory proteins.

4. Antisense strategies. This term has been used to describe nucleic acids which base pair to complementary viral RNA strands with the subsequent formation of a double stranded molecule. This binding may interfere with viral transcription as well as binding to viral and cellular factors.

5. Ribozymes are RNA molecules which are able to bind to and cleave specific RNA target sequences. Theoretically, inhibition of viral replication might be achieved by cleaving highly conserved areas in the HIV genome, such as RRE and TAR.

6. Virus-inducible "suicide genes". Certain genes such as the thymidine kinase gene from herpes simplex virus can be expressed in human cells under the control of HIV promoters. Upon HIV transactivation these genes are expressed. By administering acyclovir, the infected cells can be eliminated due to production of a phosphorylated (toxic) metabolite of acyclovir by the thymidine kinase. Alternatively, other genes which encode for directly toxic products can be used, obviating the need for a prodrug.

7. Combination strategies. Interest in combination of antiviral strategies is mounting. Several studies have already suggested that synergistic or additive effects may be achieved by using simultaneous expression of more than one antiviral gene.

Viral Targets for Gene Therapy

pol *Gene*

Ribozymes with different *pol* targets have been described. Yu and colleagues constructed a hairpin ribozyme targeted to cleave a conserved region in the *pol* gene. T cells transduced with a retroviral construct encoding this ribozyme gene exhibited significant inhibition of different strains of HIV. Greater protection was shown when the ribozyme expression was driven by a pol III promoter as compared to a pol II promoter.[4]

Reverse Transcriptase

The enzyme reverse transcriptase (RT) has been successfully inhibited by pharmacologic means using both nucleoside and nonnucleoside analogs. In addition, true "intracellular immunization" against HIV has been accomplished by intracellular expression of antibody fragments directed against RT.[5] Cells expressing the antibody fragments were resistant to infection with laboratory and clinical isolates of HIV-1 and HIV-2. The potential advantage of this approach is that it inhibits HIV replication prior to viral integration into the host genome, thereby allowing possible resolution of the infected state.[5]

Another method is being developed for inhibiting RT by using antisense oligonucleotides. Results indicate that antisense oligonucleotides to the U5 region of the viral RNA inhibit RT activity in vitro.[6] Studies on the efficacy of this approach in cells have not yet been published.

Integrase

In order for the reverse transcribed viral genome to be transcribed, it must be integrated into the genome of the host cell. After transportation to the cell nucleus the HIV DNA is inserted into the host cell DNA by a viral integrase, an enzyme which is encoded within the *pol* gene. This reaction is dissimilar to any reaction known to be involved in the normal functioning of the host cell, which makes this enzyme an attractive target for viral inhibition.[7] Inhibition of integrase expression has been accomplished in *Escherichia coli* by using a specific ribozyme molecule which recognizes a GUC sequence in the integrase RNA.[8] Single-chain variable antibody fragments which bind to different domains in the integrase have also been identified and expressed intracellularly in both T cell lines and peripheral blood mononuclear cells.[9] Furthermore, it was shown that expression of the antibody fragments specifically neutralized the enzyme prior to integration, rendering the cells resistant to productive HIV infection.[9]

Tat and TAR

The Tat protein is an attractive target for antiviral therapy, because it is a potent transactivator of HIV-1 gene expression, an effect which occurs by high-efficiency binding of the protein to the transactivation response element (TAR). This binding promotes HIV-1 LTR activation.[10,11] In order to suppress this transcriptional activation several approaches have been taken, including transdominant Tat mutants,[12-15] antisense to *tat*[16-18] and TAR,[19] and antisense Tat tRNA,[20] RNA TAR decoys,[21-29] and ribozymes which target *tat*.[16,30]

The first report of Tat transdominant mutants by Green and colleagues in 1989[13] demonstrated that HIV LTR-driven expression could be suppressed by transdominant mutants. Recent development of other constitutively expressed mutants in the transactivation region of Tat has confirmed the ability of these molecules to inhibit replication and reactivation of HIV in cell lines.[12] However this strategy has so far not been studied in primary T cells.

Sullenger and colleagues demonstrated that T cells can be rendered less susceptible to HIV replication by overexpressing TAR RNA decoys.[22] By mutagenesis they were able to show that nucleotide changes that disrupt the stem structure abolished the ability of the molecule to inhibit viral replication. They suggested that the mechanism of action of the TAR decoys involved sequestration of transactivation protein complexes consisting of Tat-TAR bound to additional cellular factors.[21] However, despite antiviral effects in selected cell clones, this strategy was fairly ineffective in bulk cell lines and primary CD4+ lymphocytes.[23] Due to concerns that constitutive expression might be deleterious to the cells, an approach where the presence of Tat induces the production of TAR decoys through LTR activation has been studied and shown to be effective in cell lines.[25] This approach has even been modified further by constructing a LTR-regulated TAR decoy which also contains a *gag*-specific ribozyme.[26] Results from challenge experiments in T cell lines suggests that a 99% suppression of both HIV-1 and SIV replication may be achieved.[26] A potential problem with all RNA decoys is a relatively short half-life due to action of endonucleases. It has been shown that stability of the decoys can be improved dramatically by using circular RNA, such as TAR RNA[27] and these circular compounds can inhibit Tat-activated HIV transcription.[29]

A comparison of antisense to *tat* and a ribozyme which targets the *tat* gene has revealed that the antisense strategy may be more effective.[16] Furthermore, an adeno-associated virus (AAV) vector encoding antisense sequences the to TAR RNA and the poly-adenylation signal has recently been studied in human hemopoietic and nonhemopoietic cell lines. Cells expressing the antisense sequences showed greater than 99% reduction in infectious HIV-1 production and no cellular toxicity was detected.[19] Since AAV is a non-pathogenic virus that does not recombine with HIV-1 and can transduce diverse cells, it may be an attractive target for clinical trials of gene therapy. However, demonstration of inhibition of HIV in primary cells using AAV has not yet been published. On the other hand, transduction of CD34+ hematopoietic progenitor cells with a retroviral vector encoding anti-*tat* gene has been shown to yield T cell and macrophage progeny which exhibit resistance to HIV.[18] Ribozymes which target the translational initiation region of *tat* have been designed and shown to be effective against laboratory strains of HIV in transfection experiments.[30]

Rev and RRE

The binding of Rev to the RRE is an essential trigger for viral production. Numerous approaches have therefore been taken to inhibit this binding and the subsequent nuclear export of unspliced mRNA. Transdominant Rev mutants,[31-39] chimeric Rev molecules which inhibit nuclear export of RNA,[40] antisense RRE sequences,[41-43] RNA decoys (Fig. 2.1),[28,44-48] ribozymes which selectively cut the RRE and intracellular antibodies which bind to Rev[49-52] have all been used. The first transdominant Rev mutant was developed in 1989 by Malim and colleagues.[31] Subsequently a number of studies have been published, demonstrating efficacy of transdominant Rev mutants in T cell lines and, more importantly, in primary T cells challenged with primary HIV isolates.[32-36,39] Currently, a phase I clinical trial in AIDS patients is underway, where the safety of administering lymphocytes expressing the mutant RevM10 is being studied.[37,38]

A novel approach for inhibiting the nuclear export of viral RNA by blocking Rev function was recently studied. A chimeric protein was generated, consisting of the wild-type Rev protein covalently linked to a mutated NS1 protein of the Influenza A virus, which inhibits nuclear resistance to breakthrough growth of virus for up to 5 weeks.[43]

Another approach to achieving Rev inhibition is to overexpress the RRE target sequence (Fig. 2.1). Lee and colleagues demonstrated that overexpression of a 45-nucleotide transcript to stem loops IIA and IIB in the RRE, expressed as a chimeric tRNA-RRE transcript, suppressed HIV in more than 90% of expressing T cells.[45] However, due to concerns that viral RNA sequences may bind and interfere with the function of essential cellular factors, a "minimal" 13 nucleotide RNA decoy corresponding to the authentic Rev binding domain has been constructed and demonstrated to confer resistance to HIV replication in T cell lines[46] as well as primary T cells.[48] Transient protection has also been shown in T cells transduced with AAV vectors expressing RRE decoys.[47] Recently, CD34+ cells have been transduced with this minimal 13 nt RRE decoy. The macrophage progeny of the committed progenitor cells were challenged with HIV and shown to be resistant to replication of macrophage-tropic strains of HIV.[44]

True intracellular immunization against Rev has also been studied by expressing an anti-Rev single-chain antibody (sFv) which inhibits HIV-1 replication in human cells.[49-51] In addition, it has been shown that the antibody is localized in the cytoplasm where it probably exerts its effects by sequestering the wild-type Rev[50] and accelerating its degeneration.[52] Both SFv and RRE decoys delivered to primary T cells and alveolar macrophages by adeno-associated virus (AAV) vector have been shown to effectively inhibit infection with both clinical and laboratory isolates, including a multidrug-resistant isolate. Moreover, the combination of both antiviral strategies seems to be synergistic.[53] A clinical trial has been proposed based on these findings (Table 2.1).

A ribozyme which targets the *rev/env* coding region of HIV has been tested in T cells. This construct protected the T cells from selected strains of HIV.[54] Furthermore, ribozymes targeting the *tat* and *rev* genes of HIV have been successfully used for temporary HIV inhibition in T cell lines.[30,55]

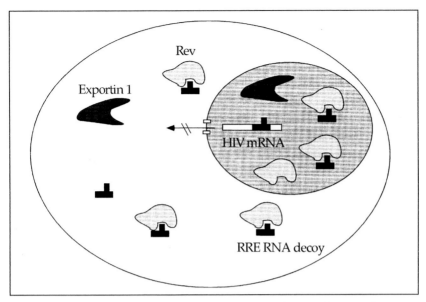

Fig. 2.1. Schematic representation of inhibition of Rev function by RNA decoys. By overexpressing the RRE sequence, the Rev protein is competitively inhibited. Similarly, the export of HIV RNA can be inhibited by using dominant negative Rev proteins.

Nef Function

The Nef protein, an early gene product which is important for maintenance of high viral loads and the development of AIDS,[56] functions to downregulate CD4+ and MHC-I expression on infected cells through endocytosis, thus evading the protective effect of CTLs.[57-59] Further evidence reinforcing the importance of this gene product has come from Deacon and colleagues, who followed 6 HIV infected individuals that were infected by the same donor by blood transfusion. These individuals have remained asymptomatic with very low viral loads for 10-14 years despite being HIV positive. Virus from all these patients have deletions in the *nef* gene, probably rendering the virus less pathogenic.[60]

Antisense oligonucleotides and ribozymes have been used to target a conserved 14 nucleotide region in the *nef* gene, demonstrating effective inhibition both in peripheral blood mononuclear cells and T cell lines.[61] Administration of Nef-specific CTLs has been described in one patient at the National Institutes of Health (Protocol 92-1-0035),[62] but minimal effects were observed from therapy.

Table 2.1. Summary of clinical protocols for gene therapy to combat HIV that have been assigned an NIH number.

NIH#	Investigators	Classification	Transduction	Target Cell	Gene	Vector	#Pts approved #Pts treated
9202-017	Greenberg, P Riddell, S	Phase I	ex vivo	CD8+ PBLCs allo- or autologous CTLs	HyTK[1]	Retrovirus	30 8
9206-026	Walker, R	Marking	ex vivo	syngeneic PBLCs	G1Na/Neo^R or LNL/Neo^{R2}	Retrovirus	12 6
9306-048	Galpin, J Casciato, D Merritt, J	Phase I	in vivo	autologous muscle cells	HIV-IT(V) or HIV-IIIB env[7]	Retrovirus	? 21
9306-049	Nabel, GJ	Phase I	ex vivo	autologous CD4+ PBLCs	pLJRevM10 pLJdltaRevM10 tar/RevM10 RSV-tar/deltaRevM10[4]	Retrovirus or particle-mediated	12 4
9309-057	Wong-Staal, F Poeschla, E Looney, D	Phase I	ex vivo	autologous CD4+ PBLCs	pJT-HR[5] (hairpin ribozyme)	Retrovirus	6 0

[1]Title: Phase I study to evaluate the safety of cellular adoptive immunotherapy using genetically modified CD8+ HIV-specific T cells in HIV seropositive individuals.

[2]Title: A study of the safety and survival of the adoptive transfer of genetically marked syngeneic lymphocytes in HIV infected identical twins.

[3]Title: A preliminary study to evaluate the safety and biologic effects of murine retroviral vector encoding HIV-1 genes (HIV-IT(V)) in asymptomatic subjects infected with HIV-1.

[4]Title: A molecular genetic intervention for AIDS—effects of a transdominant negative form of Rev.

[5]Title: A phase I clinical trial to evaluate the safety and effects in HIV-1 infected humans of autologous lymphocytes transduced with a ribozyme

NIH#	Investigators	Classification	Transduction	Target Cell	Gene	Vector	#Pts approved #Pts treated
9312-062	Haubrich, R Merritt, J	Phase I-II	in vivo	autologous muscle cells	HIV-IT(V)	Retrovirus	25
9403-069	Walker, R	Phase I-II	ex vivo	syngeneic CD8+ PBLCs	HIV-IIIB env[6] CD4 zeta chimeric T cell receptor[7]	Retrovirus	43, 2
9503-103	Morgan, R Walker, R	Phase I	ex vivo	anti-CD3 and IL-2 primed syngeneic CD4+ PBLCs	G1RevTdSv or GCRTdSN (TAR) and LNL6/Neo[R] or G1Na/Neo[R 8]	Retrovirus	8 0
9503-105	Parenti, D Haubrich, R Frame, P Powderly, W Loveless, M Merritt, J	Phase II	in vivo	autologous muscle cells	HIV-IT(V) HIV-IIIB env[9]	Retrovirus	190 124
9506-112	Marasco, WA	Phase I	ex vivo	autologous CD4+ PBLCs	SFv 105[10]	NA	NA
9504-113	Conant, M Lang, W Merritt, J	Phase I/II	in vivo	autologous muscle cells	HIV-IT(V) HIV-IIIB env[11]	Retrovirus	NA
9508-117	Rosenblatt, JD	Phase I	ex vivo	autologous CD34+ cells	"anti-HIV ribozyme" [12]	Retrovirus	NA
9508-119	Riddell, S	Phase I	ex vivo	allogeneic CD8+ CTLs	HyTK[13]	Retrovirus	NA

[6]Title: An open label, phase I/II clinical trial to evaluate the safety and biological activity of HIV-IT(V) (HIV-1IIIB env/retroviral vector) in HIV-1 infected subjects.

[7]Title: A phase I/II pilot study of the safety of the adoptive transfer of syngeneic gene-modified cytotoxic T-lymphocytes in HIV-infected identical twins.

[8]Title: Gene therapy for AIDS using retroviral mediated gene transfer to deliver HIV-1 antisense TAR and transdominant Rev protein genes to syngeneic lymphocytes in HIV infected identical twins.

[9]Title: A repeat dose safety and efficacy study of HIV-IT(V) in HIV-1 infected subjects with greater than or equal to 100 CD4+ T cells and no AIDS defining symptoms.

[10]Title: Intracellular antibodies against HIV-1 envelope protein for AIDS gene therapy.

[11]Title: A randomized, double blinded, phase I/II dosing study to evaluate the safety and optimal CTL inducing dosage of HIV-IT(V) in preselected HIV-1 infected

[12]Title: A phase I trial of autologous CD34+ hematopoietic progenitor cells transduced with an anti-HIV-1 ribozyme.

[13]Title: Phase I study to evaluate the safety of cellular adoptive immunotherapy using autologous unmodified and genetically modified CD8+ HIV-specific T cells in HIV seropositive individuals.subjects.

Table 2.1. (Continued)

NIH#	Investigators	Classification	Transduction	Target Cell	Gene	Vector	#Pts approved #Pts treated
9510-131	Connick, E Deeks, SG	Phase II	ex vivo	autologous CD4+ PBLCs	CD4 zeta chimeric T cell receptor[14]	Retrovirus	NA
9511-134	Gilbert, MJ Riddell, S Greenberg, PD Appelbaum, FR Spack, DH Coombs, RW Corey, L Kohn, DB Gooley, T	Phase I	ex vivo	autologous CD4+ PBLCs	poly TAR and RRE-poly TAR RNA decous[15]	Retrovirus	NA
9512-141	Pomerantz, RJ	Phase I	ex vivo	autologous CD4+ PBLCs	anti-Rev SFv antibody[16]	Retrovirus	NA
9602-147	Kohn, DB	Phase I	ex vivo	autologous CD34+ cells	RRE RNA decoy[17]	Retrovirus	NA

[14] Title: A randomized, controlled, phase II study of the activity and safety of autologous CD4-zeta gene-modified T cells in HIV-infected patients.

[15] Title: Phase I study to evaluate the safety and in vivo persistence of adoptively transferred autologous CD4+ T cells genetically modified to resist HIV replication.

[16] Title: Intracellular immunization against HIV-1 infection using an anti-Rev single chain variable fragment (SFv).

[17] Title: Transduction of CD34+ cells from the bone marrow of HIV-1 infected children: Comparative marking by an RRE decoy.

5' Leader Sequence (U5)

Ribozymes are RNA molecules that recognize and cleave specific sequences. Hairpin ribozymes which target the HIV-1 5' leader sequence[63,64] have by some authors been shown to inhibit HIV-1 in T cell lines,[65-67] whereas others have been unable to demonstrate antiviral effects.[28] Primary lymphocytes expressing this ribozyme have been shown to be protected from HIV replication.[68] Theoretically, all viral RNAs could be susceptible to the action of this ribozyme, since it is the leader which links the coding sequence of the mRNA to its cap structure. Therefore, the capless RNAs cannot be translated into proteins. Early work with these ribozymes has recently been extended to CD34+ cells from fetal cord blood which were transduced with a retroviral vector carrying the same ribozyme gene. Subsequently, macrophage-like cells grown from the CD34+ cells were shown to resist infection by a macrophage-tropic isolate of HIV.[69]

gag Function

The products of the *gag* gene exist in a highly multimerized form in the mature HIV virions. Therefore, it has been proposed that they may represent an attractive target for the generation of transdominant mutants.[70] A number of Gag negative mutants have been generated that can interfere with the production of infectious viral particles. Cells that expressed high levels of such negative Gag mutants had an impaired ability to support HIV replication when challenged with a wild-type virus, due to a negative effect on a late step in the viral life cycle, concomitant with or subsequent to viral assembly.[70] Other methods of *gag*-suppression have been studied, such as antisense sequences complementary to the 5' leader-*gag* region of HIV.[71,72] In T cell lines expressing the antisense sequence, HIV replication was inhibited for 10-20 days. However, despite stable expression of the protective sequence, the antiviral effect was not lasting.[72] However, by expressing a longer anti-*gag* sequence (1 kbp), a more effective and durable suppression in HIV replication has been demonstrated in primary CD4+ lymphocytes.[73] Ribozymes targeted to HIV-1 *gag* transcripts have been developed and transfected into cell lines.[74] Subsequent challenge with HIV revealed cleavage of *gag* RNA and substantial reduction of p24 production. Importantly, the ribozyme expression had no effect on cell replication and viability.

Nucleocapsid Protein

The HIV-1 nucleocapsid protein (p7NC) contains two highly conserved motifs which are coordinated to zinc, termed zinc fingers. This protein has important functions, both early in HIV infection as processed p7NC, as well as late in infection, where it exists as a precursor polyprotein which mediates packaging of viral genomic RNA into progeny virions.[75] Although no gene therapy studies which affect the p7NC have been published to date, it may be an ideal candidate for transdominant mutant or ribozyme-mediated strategies, since it is mutationally intolerant and resistant mutants have not been detected.[75]

gp120 and gp41

Cells that are infected with HIV express gp120 on the cell membrane. The expression of these viral envelope proteins has prompted investigators to design novel gene delivery vectors with tropism for the infected cells. By pseudotyping rabies virus with CD4 and CXCR-4, Mebation and co-workers were able to specifically target HIV infected cells.[76] Schnell et al similarly constructed a recombinant vesicular stomatitis virus which expressed CD4 and CXCR-4, thus targeting gp120/gp41-expressing cells (Fig. 2.2). This virus selectively propagated in and killed HIV infected cells, but was unable to infect normal cells.[77]

Intracellular immunization by using a intracellular single chain antibody to the gp120 (sFv105) has been studied in eukaryotic cells.[78] It is designed to react with the nascent folded envelope protein (gp160) within the endoplasmic reticulum, to prevent cleavage to gp120 and inhibit subsequent transit of the envelope antibody complex to the cell surface. In cell lines that express the antibody it has been shown to be retained in the endoplasmic reticulum, where it inhibits processing of the envelope precursor and subsequent syncytia formation. In addition, it was demonstrated that the infectivity of the cells expressing the antibody was substantially reduced.[78] However, the effect was relatively short-lived, since the viral replication was only delayed temporarily (5 days).

Multitarget ribozymes which target several different sites in the gp120 region of the HIV RNA have recently been developed. Some of these constructs target up to nine different conserved regions in the RNA (nonaribozymes).[79] Results from cotransfection experiments in cell lines indicate that antiviral activity can be substan-

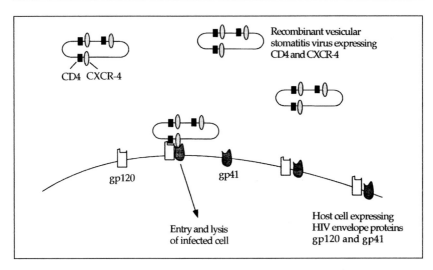

Fig. 2.2. Selective targeting of HIV-infected cells. By expressing CD4 and CXCR-4 on a recombinant viral particle, cells which express the HIV envelope glycoproteins gp120 and gp41 can be selectively infected and destroyed, whereas uninfected cells are not affected.

tially increased by using several hammerheads with catalytic activity on the same molecule (see below, combinations of antiviral strategies).

Protease

The viral protease which belongs to the family of aspartyl proteases is essential for the life cycle of HIV by cleaving the Gag-pol polyprotein into structural proteins as well as the virion enzymes. The recent success in pharmacologic inhibition of the enzyme has sparked interest in this enzyme and its inhibition by using gene therapy. Transdominant mutant protease has been constructed and shown to prevent protease activation and virion maturation.[80] Junker and co-workers showed that T cell lines which constitutively expressed the mutant protein had dramatically reduced HIV replication when compared to cells expressing the wild-type protein. Furthermore, this approach was also shown to be effective against protease-resistant isolates.[81] Another approach to inhibit the protease through competitive inhibition has been taken by Serio and colleagues, who created a chimeric Vpr molecule which also contained a protease cleavage site[82] (see below, accessory proteins).

The Vpr, Vif and Vpu Accessory Proteins

An attractive target for gene therapy in the future could involve the nuclear localization signal (NLS) of the Vpr or matrix proteins, both of which mediate transfer of the preintegration complex to the cell nucleus,[83] enabling HIV to infect nondividing cells.[84-86] In addition the Vpr protein also arrests the infected cells in G_2 of the cell cycle, thus increasing viral production of each cell.[86] The protein furthermore has a role in virion incorporation and has specificity for the HIV viral particle. The specificity of Vpr for the viral particle can be used to deliver antiviral elements interfering with virus maturation.[87] A recent report from Serio and colleagues describes the use of chimeric Vpr proteins containing HIV-specific protease cleavage sites added to the C terminus of the Vpr. Interestingly, the chimeric Vpr containing the cleavage junction from p24 and p2 completely abolished virus infectivity.[82] The authors suggested that the mechanism of inhibition was by overwhelming protease activity, since the cleavage site of the 24/2 serves as a regulator for the sequential processing of the Gag precursor.[82] No gene therapy approaches to inhibit Vif and Vpu have yet been published.

Packaging Sequence ψ

The ψ packaging sequence is required for efficient packaging of HIV RNA into virions.[88,89] Deletion of 19 nucleotides encompassing ψ between the 5' LTR and the *gag* initiation codon results in a markedly replication-attenuated virus.[88] Antisense sequences to ψ, as well as ribozymes which specifically cleave the ψ sequence, have been shown to render T cell clones less susceptible to HIV replication.[90]

HIV-Induced Suicide Genes

A novel approach to selectively kill HIV-infected cells involves the introduction of suicide genes to the genome of the cell. As an example the herpes simplex Type 1 thymidine kinase gene (HSV-TK), under the transcriptional control of HIV-1 LTR[91] or modified HIV-2 promoters,[92] has been used to inhibit HIV. Upon infection with HIV the HSV-TK gene is transcribed and in turn phosphorylates acyclovir, which is added to the medium, to its toxic metabolite. This approach has been shown to work in vitro; spread of HIV was halted in cell cultures which were infected with HIV upon addition of acyclovir[91] or gancyclovir[92] in concentrations routinely achieved in the clinical setting. Similar studies have been conducted using replication-defective adenoviral vectors.[93] Other genes can be used to selectively kill HIV-infected cells, for instance diphtheria toxin A (DT-A) under the transcriptional regulation of the Tat and Rev proteins.[94,95] Another method to selectively kill HIV-infected cells has been described using a hybrid molecule of the human CD4 and a modified version of the *Pseudomonas* exotoxin A (CD4-PE40).[96] This molecule is designed to bind specifically to HIV-infected cells by CD4-gp120 interaction at the cell surface. After this binding the receptor-ligand complex is internalized and the exotoxin inhibits protein synthesis, leading to cell death. CD4-PE40 has been studied extensively in cell lines infected with laboratory strains of HIV where efficacy has been demonstrated. However, in the presence of primary isolates the CD4-PE40 is less active, since continuous presence of the molecule was required to inhibit HIV replication.[96]

The *vhs* (shutoff) gene in herpes simplex virus encodes a protein which nonspecifically accelerates the degradation of mRNA, thus inhibiting protein synthesis. When the Vhs protein was expressed from the HIV LTR promoter, HIV replication was inhibited more than 44,000-fold when compared to a nonfunctional mutant.[97]

Cellular Targets for Gene Therapy

CD4

It has been known since 1984 that the lymphocyte surface marker CD4 is essential for virus entry into host cells and that monoclonal antibodies against CD4 can inhibit infection by HIV.[98] This led to the hypothesis that CD4 could be used as an antiviral agent against HIV. Initially, encouraging results were seen which demonstrated that soluble CD4 (sCD4) could neutralize laboratory isolates of HIV in vitro. This early enthusiasm was tempered by the sobering finding that most primary isolates need much higher (200-2700-fold higher) doses of sCD4 to achieve a neutralizing effect.[99] However, it is theoretically possible that immunization with sCD4 may induce an anti-CD4 antibody response which possesses an anti-HIV activity, as seen in a simian animal model.[100,101]

Another potential therapeutic option involves expression of intracellular CD4, mutated to contain a specific retention signal for the endoplasmic reticulum.[102] By expression of this molecule, secretion of gp120 and surface expression of gp120/gp41 was inhibited in cell lines. This intracellular trap led to disappearance of infected cells over a period of two months.[103] However, the effects of this antiviral strategy in primary T cells and primary HIV isolates have not been published.

Chemokine Receptors Ccr-5 and Cxcr-4

Recently, remarkable progress has been made in the search for cellular coreceptors for HIV. A family of chemokine receptors, CCR-5 and CXCR-4 have recently been identified as the HIV coreceptors.[104-109] The chemokines are important in regulation of phagocyte and lymphocyte recruitment.[110] It has been shown that the β-chemokines MIP-1α, MIP-1β and RANTES can inhibit primary strains of HIV, probably through competitive inhibition of the coreceptor.[111,112] The fact that some individuals seem to be less susceptible to primary HIV infection has recently merged with the area of chemokine receptor research. Liu and colleagues have now shown that some of these individuals that remain uninfected despite multiple exposures to HIV have a homozygous defect in CCR-5, resulting in a severely truncated protein which can not be detected at the cell surface.[113] Furthermore, combined data from several large AIDS cohort studies has recently revealed that the frequency of the deletion *CCR5* heterozygotes is significantly higher among patients with HIV infection who have survived for more than 10 years.[114] The CCR-5 receptor is therefore an obvious target for various methods of pharmacologic intervention. Apart from pharmacologic inhibition, this molecule could become an attractive target for gene therapy. Resistance to HIV could possibly be achieved by using gene-modified stem-cells encoding a ribozyme molecule which could make them phenotypically homozygous for the deletion. Yang and colleagues have recently created a phenotypic knockout in lymphocytes by expressing a modified chemokine in the endoplasmic reticulum of the cells. This strategy blocked the surface expression of the CCR-5 molecule, and the cells were found to be resistant to infection by macrophage-tropic isolates of HIV.[115]

NF-κB

The cellular transcription factor nuclear factor-κB (NF-κB), originally described in 1987 by Nabel and Baltimore,[116] has been shown to regulate viral transcription of HIV-1 through two binding sites in the LTR region of HIV. In most inactive cell types the factor exists as a cytoplasmic complex bound to the inhibitor IκB. However, mitogen stimulation and infection with some viruses results in release of NF-κB from IκB and translocation to the nucleus.[117,118] Through its contribution to Tat-mediated transactivation, NF-κB can further increase levels of early spliced HIV RNA.[116,119]

Based on these facts, a relative increase in IκB expression could therefore inhibit HIV transcription. Cells transfected with an IκB encoding plasmid have been shown to exhibit significant suppression in HIV replication. This effect is mediated through a posttranslational mechanism, most likely negatively regulating a cellular factor involved in Rev transactivation.[120] Furthermore, recent studies have described the generation of novel transdominant mutants of IκB that are even more effective than the wild-type IκB in suppressing HIV gene expression and multiplication.[121]

Eukaryotic Initiation Factor 5A

Another cellular cofactor of Rev, eukaryotic initiation factor 5A (eIF-5A) has been identified as a cellular cofactor of Rev.[122] Bevec and colleagues described two nonfunctional mutants which retained their binding capacity for the Rev-RRE complex. When these mutants were expressed in human T cells and infected with HIV, replication was inhibited due to suppressive effects on Rev-mediated transactivation and nuclear export.[123] These results have been supported by subsequent studies in primary T cells.[124]

Interferons and RBP9-27

Interferons (IFN) have been demonstrated to suppress HIV replication, affecting various stages in the viral life cycle.[125-127] A cellular factor, RNA binding protein 9-27 (RBP9-27), induced by IFN-α and IFN-γ, has been identified and demonstrated to antagonize Rev function.[127] This suggests that inhibition of HIV might be accomplished by stimulation of a cellular IFN-mediated defense system, possibly by interfering with the Rev-RRE posttranscriptional regulatory pathway.

Peripheral blood mononuclear cells isolated from HIV-1-infected individuals show diminished production of IFN-α after exposure to viruses.[127] It has therefore been postulated that enhancement of autocrine IFN synthesis might suppress HIV replication. Cells transduced with a retrovirus encoding the human IFN-β gene have been demonstrated to resist entry of a wide variety of retroviruses, including HIV.[128] This work has been extended to primary T cells. Transduced lymphocytes from healthy seronegative donors as well as asymptomatic HIV infected individuals have been shown to suppress HIV replication.[129] In addition, survival advantage and enrichment for cells expressing the IFN-β gene following challenge with HIV has also been demonstrated by the same authors.[129] These encouraging findings are supported by preliminary results from a clinical study which suggest that a combination of IL-2 and IFN-α, when given intravenously, may suppress HIV titers in patients.[130]

Other Cellular Cofactors

Although inhibition of the following cellular cofactors has not been studied in the context of gene therapy, they constitute potential targets which may become amiable to genetic manipulation in the future.

1. AP-2. This is a cellular cofactor which binds to the HIV LTR and modulates HIV enhancer function.[131] This factor binds to the site between the NFκB elements, and mutations which disrupt the AP-2 binding site have been shown to result in lower basal level of transcription in Jurkat cells. It has therefore been suggested that AP-2 could function as a repressor of transcription of viral and cellular genes in stimulated cells by antagonizing NFκB binding.[131]

2. Sp1. The cellular transcription factor Sp1 has three sites in the HIV LTR in close proximity to the two binding sites for NFκB.[132] Recent findings suggest that this juxtaposition of DNA-binding sites promotes a specific protein interaction between Sp1 and NF-κB, and that this interaction is required for HIV transcriptional activation.[133]

3. Rev cofactors. Exportin 1 (crm1p) is a nuclear export protein which has been shown to bind to the nuclear export signal of Rev and transport singly-spliced and unspliced HIV RNA to the cytoplasm.[134-136] In addition, the Rev/Rex activation domain-binding (RAB) protein binds to the activation domain of Rev in HIV-1 when Rev is assembled onto RRE. Overexpression of this protein results in increase in HIV-1 replication.[137] The feasibility of inhibiting these cellular factors to suppress HIV replication has not been studied.

4. SF2/ASF. This factor is a member of the SR family of splicing factors and has been shown to bind to a subregion of the RRE in a Rev-dependent manner, inhibiting viral RNA splicing and thus enhancing production of singly-spliced and unspliced viral RNA needed for viral propagation.[138] It has also been shown that expression of high levels of SF2/AST inhibits Rev function and HIV replication.[138]

Combinations of Antiviral Strategies

Although most studies have so far only focused on single antiviral genes to assess their efficacy in cell cultures, combinations of antiviral elements in a single vector is likely to confer added benefit.

Ribozyme-RNA Decoy Combinations

A combination of ribozymes and RNA decoys has recently been described. A ribozyme with an RRE or TAR sequence coupled to the stem loop of each ribozyme was shown to exhibit dual function in vitro.[139] A combination of TAR decoys and *gag*-specific ribozymes has been shown to suppress HIV and SIV in T cell lines.[26] Another chimeric molecule consisting of an RRE RNA decoy fused with a ribozyme directed at the HIV-1 U5 sequence has been constructed. Subsequent challenge of T cells transduced with this construct revealed much greater protection in cells expressing the chimeric construct as compared to the ribozyme molecule alone.[140] A triple-copy vector encoding the U5 ribozyme, ribozyme against the *env/rev* region and RRE decoy has recently been shown to be confer T cells an even higher level of resistance against diverse clades of HIV-1.[2]

Transdominant Mutant Combinations

A combination of two transdominant mutant proteins seems to increase HIV suppression. When expressed simultaneously, Tat and Rev transdominant mutants resulted in additive or even synergistic inhibition of HIV when compared to the Rev mutant alone.[141] This paradigm also seems to apply to other combinations, such as TAR-decoys combined with either dominant mutants of the *gag* gene or *gag* antisense sequences.[24]

Antisense Combinations

Dual inhibition by antisense oligonucleotides to both the TAR and the polyadenylation signal has been shown to reduce the production of infectious HIV by more than 99% in cell lines.[19] Similarly, expression of multitargeting *tat/rev* antisense sequences has been shown to result in stable resistance to HIV in monocytic cells.[17]

Intracellular Antibodies with RNA Decoys

Recent data from primary T cells and alveolar macrophages shows that combination of anti-Rev single chain immunoglobulin (SFv) and RRE RNA decoy delivered by AAV vectors results in synergistic inhibition of both laboratory and clinical isolates of HIV-1.[53] Although proviral sequences could be detected following challenge with HIV, viral production (p24) was 3 logs lower in the cells harboring the combination.

Multitarget Ribozymes

A novel approach to HIV inhibition has been taken by Chen and colleagues, who constructed several novel multitarget ribozymes with variable numbers of hammerhead motifs (mono-, di-, tetra-, penta-, and nonaribozymes), each of which was targeted to cleave HIV-1 *env* RNA at up to nine conserved sites.[79] Activity of the ribozyme construct roughly paralleled the number of catalytic motifs on the molecules. In cotransfection experiments in cell lines, HIV replication was found to be inhibited as measured by p24 production and syncytia formation. Moreover, a dramatic reduction of the *env* transcripts was shown in cells expressing the nonaribozymes. Another modification of ribozymes has recently been described, using so-called "shotgun" ribozymes against HIV.[142] These are multiple ribozymes, flanked by cis-acting ribozymes at both their 3' and 5' ends. Upon transcription multiple ribozyme molecules are trimmed at their 3' and 5' ends, resulting in release of multiple independent ribozymes, each of which can be targeted differently. Furthermore, it has been shown that RNA decoys (RRE and TAR) can also be added to the cis-acting ribozymes, further enhancing the antiviral activity of this technique by sequestering Tat and Rev in vitro.[139] However, despite promising results in vitro these ribozymes have still not been studied in vivo and are currently not usable in retroviral vectors, but alternatively an AAV vector might be used.[142]

Other Approaches

Genetic Immunotherapy

While the pivotal importance of viral replication in HIV pathogenesis cannot be ignored, several studies suggest that the immune system, particularly CD8+ cells, has an important role in suppressing HIV replication.[143-149] It has been shown that increased TH1 responses (IL-2) correlate with increased cell-mediated immunity against HIV, whereas an increase in cytokines from TH2 cells (IL-4, IL-10) may suppress the CTL responses against HIV.[144] A novel approach to enhancing CTL activity against HIV-infected T cells has been taken by Walker and colleagues.[62] They have constructed a gene encoding a chimeric receptor with domains from an HIV-specific molecule (CD4, which binds gp120) and a T cell receptor, CD3 ζ (zeta) chain. It is thought that the CD3 ζ chain is the signal transducer triggering the cytotoxic activity of CD8+ cells, and therefore this chimeric receptor could recognize HIV infected cells and immediately initiate a cytotoxic response (Fig. 2.3).[150] It has been shown in vitro that these gene-modified cells exhibit cytolytic activity against target cells expressing gp120 (*env* gene) at effector to target ratios as low as 0.3:1.[62] An open label comparative clinical protocol has been proposed where HIV infected individuals who possess a seronegative syngeneic twin would receive genetically modified ex vivo expanded CD8+ T lymphocytes (Table 2.1).

Site-Specific Recombination

A molecular strategy to excise proviral DNA from cells infected with HIV-1 and render the cells free from virus is an attractive antiviral strategy if a mechanism for specific removal of viral genes from infected cells can be designed. Flowers et al studied the Cre-*loxP* recombination system of bacteriophage P1, which catalyzes site-specific recombination. They demonstrated that T cell lines transformed with the Cre expression vector supported substantially less HIV replication when challenged with the recombinant HIV-1^{lox} clone and evidence for the excised products was demonstrated.[151]

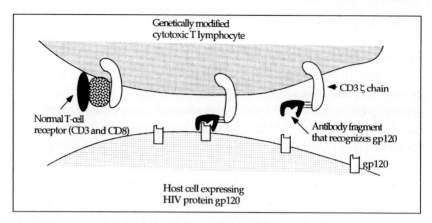

Fig. 2.3. Construction of a chimeric HIV-specific receptor and expression in cytotoxic T cells. Antibody domains from heavy- and light-chain variable regions that recognize gp120 are connected to the CD3ζ (zeta) chain, which is believed to be the signal transducer triggering cytotoxic activity of CD8+ cells. Therefore, on contact with an HIV infected cell the transmembrane CD3ζ chain can initiate a cytotoxic response.

Clinical Protocols

Several of the gene therapy strategies described on the preceding pages have been proposed as alternative treatments for HIV infection. Clinical protocols that have been accepted or are listed by the Recombinant DNA Advisory Committee (RAC) in the USA are listed in Table 2.1.

While several clinical studies are being conducted or contemplated, only a few investigators have yet published their results. Results from a small phase I study on transdominant Rev mutants have recently been published.[38] The fate of autologous T cells in two HIV infected patients were studied after transduction ex vivo with Rous sarcoma virus (RSV) expression plasmids by particle-mediated gene transfer.[37] The vectors coded for the transdominant mutant RevM10 and the control ΔrevM10, which does not inhibit Rev. The gene-modified cells were mixed in equal numbers and administered to the patients. By limiting dilution PCR it was shown that cells expressing RevM10 had a 4- to 5-fold selective survival advantage compared to controls, being detected for 56 days after infusion in one patient, while the control cells were undetectable within a week after treatment.

Another clinical study looked at immune restoration in HIV infected patients by administering autologous CD8+ HIV *gag*-specific cytotoxic T cells that had been modified by retroviral transduction to express a gene permitting positive and negative selection (the

HyTK fusion gene).[152] However this study was limited by the unexpected development of cytotoxic T lymphocyte responses against the novel protein, resulting in elimination of the modified cells in 5/6 patients treated.

Immune restoration through induction of specific cytotoxic T lymphocyte (CTL) responses has also been studied extensively and preliminary results recently published. Autologous fibroblasts were transduced with a amphotropic murine retroviral vector encoding for the HIV IIIB env/rev proteins and administered to HIV infected patients. An increase in CTL responses was demonstrated in 2/4 patients studied.[153] However, although the results are encouraging, the significance of this CTL response remains to be seen. Currently a phase II study is ongoing to determine the safety and immunotherapeutic potential of this retroviral "vaccine" for HIV. This multicenter study will enroll 168 patients,[154] but no results are yet available.

Conclusions and Future Prospects

Intense efforts to understand how HIV causes AIDS has resulted in significant progress in our understanding of retrovirology, cell biology and immunology. These advances have already translated into clinical benefit for HIV infected patients. Several questions remain unanswered regarding advances in combination drug therapy, such as long-term efficacy, the emergence of resistance, toxicity and cost.

Most current studies on gene therapy for HIV are in their initial stages. For example, most articles describe suppression in somewhat arbitrary systems of cell lines and laboratory isolates, a situation which is remote from clinical reality. Moreover, even experiments which utilize primary T cells and clinical HIV isolates are fraught with problems of experimental variation, as well as the short life span of T cells in culture. In addition, in vitro systems are arbitrary since they omit several factors which may be of importance in the in vivo setting, such as the effects of cell-mediated immunity.

Despite all these shortcomings there is reason for cautious optimism. In concert with our improved understanding of HIV biology, advances will be made in the design of vectors encoding for multiple antiviral genes, each inhibiting different targets. As outlined above, although several of these targets have been successfully exploited to achieve suppression in HIV replication, new viral proteins, nucleic acid sequences and cellular factors await further experiments to move us closer to a more effective and durable antiviral strategy. In addition, rapid progress in the field of stem cell biology is going to facilitate the use of durably gene-modified cells. Only time will tell whether these advances will translate into clinical benefits to patients through gene therapy. Quoting David Baltimore, who proposed the use of "intracellular immunization" to inhibit HIV in 1988: "Gene therapy is still a dream, although not a fantasy".[155]

Acknowledgments

I thank Dr. Paul R. Bohjanen for comments on the manuscript. MG is supported in part by a NATO science fellowship.

References

1. Marcel T, Grausz JD. The TMC worldwide gene therapy enrollment report end 1996. Hum Gene Ther 1997; 8:775-800.
2. Gervaix A, Li X, Kraus G, Wong-Staal F. Multigene antiviral vectors inhibit diverse human immunodeficiency virus type 1 clades. J Virol 1997; 71:3048-3053.
3. Paillard F. The use of peripheral blood hematopoietic progenitors for human immunodeficiency virus gene therapy. Hum Gene Ther 1997; 8:2170-2172.
4. Yu M, Poeschla E, Yamada O et al. In vitro and in vivo characterization of a second functional hairpin ribozyme against HIV-1. Virology 1995; 206:381-386.
5. Maciejewski JP, Weichold FF, Young NS et al. Intracellular expression of antibody fragments directed against HIV reverse transcriptase prevents HIV infection in vitro. Nature Med 1995; 1:667-673.
6. Bordier B, Helene C, Barr PJ, Litvak S, Sarih-Cottin L. In vitro effect of antisense oligonucleotides on human immunodeficiency virus type 1 reverse transcription. Nucleic Acids Res 1992; 20: 5999-6006.
7. Craigie R, Hickman AB, Engelman A. Integrase. In: Karn J, ed. HIV. Biochemistry, molecular biology and drug discovery. Vol. 2. Oxford: Oxford University Press, 1995:53-71.
8. Sioud M, Drlica K. Prevention of human immunodeficiency virus type 1 integrase expression in *Escherichia coli* by a ribozyme. Proc Natl Acad Sci USA 1991; 88:7303-7307.
9. Levy-Mintz P, Duan L, Zhang H et al. Intracellular expression of single-chain variable fragments to inhibit early stages of the viral life cycle by targeting human immunodeficiency virus type 1 integrase. J Virol 1996; 70:8821-8832.
10. Berkhout B, Silverman RH, Jeang K-T. Tat *Trans*-activates the human immunodeficiency virus through a nascent RNA target. Cell 1990; 59:273-282.
11. Selby MJ, Peterlin BM. *Trans*-Activation by HIV-1 Tat via a heterologous RNA binding protein. Cell 1990; 62:769-776.

12. Caputo A, Grossi MP, Rossi C et al. Inhibition of HIV-1 replication and reactivation from latency by tat transdominant negative mutants in the cysteine rich region. Gene Therapy 1996; 3:235-245.
13. Green M, Ishino M, Loewenstein PM. Mutational analysis of HIV-1 Tat minimal domain peptides: Identification of trans-dominant mutants that suppress HIV-LTR-driven gene expression. Cell 1989; 58:215-223.
14. Modesti N, Garcia J, Debouck C, Peterlin M, Gaynor R. Trans-dominant Tat mutants with alterations in the basic domain inhibit HIV-1 gene expression. New Biol 1991; 3:759-768.
15. Pearson L, Garcia J, Wu F, Modesti N, Nelson J, Gaynor R. A transdominant *tat* mutant that inhibits tat-induced gene expression from the human immunodeficiency virus long terminal repeat. Proc Natl Acad Sci USA 1990; 87:5079-5083.
16. Lo KMS, Biasolo MA, Dehni G, Palu G, Haseltine WA. Inhibition of replication of HIV-1 by retroviral vectors expressing *tat*-antisense and anti-*tat* ribozyme RNA. Virology 1992; 190:176-183.
17. Liu D, Donegan J, Nuovo G, Mitra D, Laurence J. Stable human immunodeficiency virus type 1 (HIV-1) resistance in transformed CD4+ monocytic cells treated with multitargeting HIV-1 antisense sequences incorporated into U1 snRNA. J Virol 1997; 71:4079-4085.
18. Rosenzweig M, Marks DF, Hempel D, Lisziewicz J, Johnson RP. Transduction of CD34+ hematopoietic progenitor cells with an *antitat* gene protects T cell and macrophage progeny from AIDS virus infection. J Virol 1997; 71:2740-2746.
19. Chatterjee S, Johnson PR, Wong KK Jr. Dual-target inhibition of HIV-1 in vitro by means of an adeno-associated virus antisense vector. Science 1992; 258:1485-1488.
20. Biasolo MA, Radelli A, Del Pup L, Franchin E, De Giuli-Morghen C, Palu G. A new antisense tRNA construct for the genetic tratment of human immunodeficiency virus type 1 infection. J Virol 1996; 70:2154-2161.
21. Sullenger BA, Gallardo HF, Ungers GE, Gilboa E. Analysis of trans-acting response decoy RNA-mediated inhibition of human immuodeficiency virus type 1 transactivation. J Virol 1991; 65: 6811-6816.
22. Sullenger BA, Gallardo HF, Ungers GE, Gilboa E. Overexpression of TAR sequences renders cells resistant to human immunodeficiency virus replication. Cell 1990; 63:601-608.
23. Lee SW, Gallardo HF, Smith C, Gilboa E. Inhibition of HIV-1 in CEM cells by a potent TAR decoy. Gene Therapy 1995; 2:377-384.
24. Lori F, Lisziewicz J, Smythe J et al. Rapid protection against human immunodeficiency virus type 1 (HIV-1) replication mediated by high efficiency nonretroviral delivery of genes interfering with HIV-1 tat and gag. Gene Therapy 1994; 1:27-31.
25. Lisziewicz J, Rappaport J, Dhar R. Tat-regulated production of multimerized TAR RNA inhibits HIV-1 gene expression. New Biol 1991; 3:82-89.

26. Lisziewics J, Sun D, Smythe J et al. Inhibition of human immuno-deficiency virus type 1 replication by regulated expression of polymeric Tat activation response RNA decoy as a strategy for gene therapy in AIDS. Proc Natl Acad Sci USA 1993; 90:8000-8004.

27. Bohjanen PR, Colvin RA, Puttarju M, Been MD, Garcia-Blanco MA. A small circular TAR RNA decoy specifically inhibits Tat-activated HIV-1 transcription. Nucleic Acids Res 1996; 24:3733-3738.

28. Good PD, Krikos AJ, Li SXL et al. Expression of small, therapeutic RNAs in human cell nuclei. Gene Ther 1997; 4:45-54.

29. Bohjanen PR, Liu Y, Garcia-Blanco MA. TAR RNA decoys inhibit Tat-activated HIV-1 transcription after preinitiation complex formation. Nucleic Acids Res 1997; 25:4481-4486.

30. Sun LQ, Wang L, Gerlach WL, Symonds G. Target sequence-specific inhibition of HIV-1 replication by ribozymes directed to *tat* RNA. Nucleic Acids Res 1995; 23:2909-2913.

31. Malim MH, Bohnlein S, Hauber J, Cullen BR. Functional dissection of the HIV-1 Rev trans-activator—derivation of a trans-dominant repressor of Rev function. Cell 1989; 58:205-214.

32. Escaich S, Kalfglou C, Plavec I, Kaushal S, Mosca JD, Bohnlein E. RevM10-mediated inhibition of HIV-1 replication in chronically infected T cells. Human Gene Ther 1995; 6:625-634.

33. Liu J, Wofferdin C, Yang ZY, Nabel GJ. Regulated expression of a dominant negative form of rev improves resistance to HIV replication in T cells. Gene Therapy 1994; 1:32-37.

34. Malim MH, Freimuth WW, Liu J et al. Stable expression of transdominant Rev protein in human T cells inhibits human immunodeficiency virus replication. J Exp Med 1992; 176:1197-1201.

35. Ragheb JA, Bressler P, Daucher M et al. Analysis of trans-dominant mutants of the HIV type 1 rev protein for their ability to inhibit rev function, HIV type 1 replication, and their use as anti-HIV gene therapeutics. AIDS Res Hum Retroviruses 1995; 11:1343-1353.

36. Wofferdin C, Yang ZY, Udaykumar et al. Nonviral and viral delivery of a human immunodeficiency virus protective gene into primary human T cells. Proc Natl Acad Sci USA 1994; 91:11581-11585.

37. Wofferdin C, Ranga U, Yang ZY, Xu L, Nabel GJ. Expression of a protective gene prolongs survival of T cells in human immunodeficiency virus-infected patients. Proc Natl Acad Sci USA 1996; 93:2889-2894.

38. Nabel GJ, Fox BA, Post L, Thompson CB, Wofferdin C. A molecular genetic intervention for AIDS-Effects of a transdominant negative form of rev. Human Gene Ther 1994; 5:79-92.

39. Plavec I, Agarwal M, Ho KE et al. High transdominant RevM10 protein levels are required to inhibit HIV-1 replication in cell lines and primary T cells: Implication for gene therapy of AIDS. Gene Ther 1997; 4:128-139.

40. Qian X, Chen Z, Zhang J, Rabson AB, Krug RM. New approach for inhibiting REV function and HIV-1 production using the influenza virus NS1 protein. Proc. Natl. Acad. Sci. USA 1996; 93:8873-8877.

41. Li G, Lisziewicz J, Sun D et al. Inhibition of Rev activity and human immunodeficiency virus type 1 replication by antisense oligodeoxynucleotide phosphothioate analogs directed against the Rev-response element. J Virol 1993; 67:6882-6888.

42. Lisziewicz J, Sun D, Klotman M, Agrawal S, Zamecnik P, Gallo R. Specific inhibition of human immunodeficiency virus type 1 replication by antisense oligonucleotides: An in vitro model for treatment. Proc Natl Acad Sci USA 1992; 89:11209-11213.

43. Sczakiel G, Oppenlander M, Rittner K, Pawlita M. Tat- and Rev-directed antisense RNA expression inhibits and abolishes replication of human immunodeficiency virus type 1: a temporal analysis. J Virol 1992; 66:5576-5581.

44. Bahner I, Kearns K, Hao Q, Smogorzewska EM, Kohn DB. Transduction of human CD34+ hematopoietic progenitor cells by a retroviral vector expressing an RRE decoy inhibits human immunodeficiency virus type 1 replication in myelomonocytic cells produced in long term culture. J Virol. 1996; 70:4352-4360.

45. Lee TC, Sullenger BA, Gallardo HF, Ungers GE, Gilboa E. Overexpression of RRE-derived sequences inhibits HIV-1 replication in CEM cells. New Biol 1992; 4:66-74.

46. Lee SW, Gallardo HF, Gilboa E, Smith C. Inhibition of Human Immunodeficiency Virus Type 1 in human T cells by a potent rev response element decoy consisting of the 13-nucleotide minimal rev-binding domain. J Virol. 1994; 68:8254-8264.

47. Smith C, Lee S-W, Wong E et al. Transient protection of human T cells from human immunodeficiency virus type 1 infection by transduction with adeno-associated viral vectors which express RNA decoys. Antiviral Res 1996; 32:99-115.

48. Gottfredsson M, Gentry T, Phillips K, Hull S, Gilboa E, Smith C. Suppression of HIV-1 replication in human T cells transduced with an RNA decoy mimicking the rev binding domain of RRE (abstr. I15), 36th Interscience Conference on Antimicrobial Agents and Chemotherapy, New Orleans, 1996. American Society for Microbiology.

49. Duan L, Zhang H, Oakes JW, Bagasra O, Pomerantz RJ. Molecular and virological effects of intracellular anti-Rev single-chain variable fragments on the expression of various human immunodeficency virus-1 strains. Human Gene Ther 1994; 5:1315-1324.

50. Duan L, Bagasra O, Laughlin MA, Oakes JW, Pomerantz RJ. Potent inhibition of human immunodeficiency virus type 1 replication by an intracellular anti-Rev single-chain antibody. Proc Natl Acad Sci USA 1994; 91:5075-5079.

51. Wu Y, Duan L, Zhu M et al. Binding of intracellular anti-rev single chain variable fragments to different epitopes of human immunodeficiency virus type 1 rev: variations in viral inhibition. J Virol 1996; 70:3290-3297.

52. Kubota S, Duan L, Furuta RA, Hatanaka M, Pomerantz RJ. Nuclear preservation and cytoplasmic degradation of human immunodeficiency virus type 1 Rev protein. J Virol 1996; 70:1282-1287.

53. Inouye RT, Du B, Boldt-Houle D et al. Potent inhibition of human immunodeficiency virus type 1 in primary T cells and alveolar macrophages by a combination anti-Rev strategy delivered in an adeno-associated virus vector. J Virol 1997; 71:4071-4078.

54. Yamada O, Kraus G, Leavitt MC, Yu M, Wong-Staal F. Activity and cleavage site specificity of an anti-HIV-1 hairpin ribozyme in human T cells. Virology 1994; 205:121-126.

55. Zhou C, Bahner IC, Larson GP, Zaia JA, Rossi JJ, Kohn DB. Inhibition of HIV-1 in human T lymphocytes by retrovirally transduced anti-*tat* and *rev* hammerhead ribozymes. Gene 1994; 149:33-39.

56. Kestler HW III, Ringler DJ, Mori K et al. Importance of the *nef* gene for maintenance of high virus loads and for development of AIDS. Cell 1991; 65:651-662.

57. Aiken C, Konner J, Landau NR, Lenburg ME, Trono D. Nef induces CD4 endocytosis: requirement for a critical dileucine motif in the membrane-proximal CD4 cytoplasmic domain. Cell 1994; 76:853-864.

58. Kerkau T, Schmitt-Landgraf R, Schimpl A, Wecker E. Down-regulation of HLA class I antigens in HIV-1-infected cells. AIDS Res Hum Retroviruses 1989; 5:613-620.

59. Schwartz O, Maréchal V, Le Gall S, Lemonnier F, Heard J-M. Endocytosis of major histocompatibility complex class I molecules is induced by the HIV-1 nef protein. Nature Med 1996; 2:338-342.

60. Deacon NJ, Tsykin A, Solomon A et al. Genomic structure of an attenuated quasi species of HIV-1 from a blood transfusion donor and recipients. Science 1995; 270:988-991.

61. Larsson S, Hotchkiss G, Su J et al. A novel ribozyme target site located in the HIV-1 *Nef* open reading frame. Virology 1996; 219:161-169.

62. Walker RE, Blease RM, Davey RT, Falloon J, Mullen C, Polis MA. A phase I/II pilot study of the safety of the adoptive transfer of syngeneic gene-modified cytotoxic T lymphocytes in HIV-infected identical twins. Human Gene Ther 1996; 7:367-400.

63. Ojwang JO, Hampel A, Looney DJ, Wong-Staal F, Rappaport J. Inhibition of human immunodeficiency virus type 1 expression by a hairpin ribozyme. Proc Natl Acad Sci USA 1992; 89:10802-10806.

64. Dropulic B, Lin NH, Martin MA, Jeang K-T. Functional characterization of a U5 ribozyme: Intracellular suppression of human immunodeficiency virus type 1 expression. J Virol 1992; 66:1432-1441.

65. Yamada O, Yu M, Yee JK, Kraus G, Looney D, Wong-Staal F. Intracellular immunization of human T cells with a hairpin ribozyme against human immunodeficiency virus type 1. Gene Therapy 1994; 1:38-45.

66. Yu M, Ojwang J, Yamada O et al. A hairpin ribozyme inhibits expression of diverse strains of human immunodeficiency virus Type 1. Proc Natl Acad Sci USA 1993; 90:6340-6344.

67. Weerasinghe M, Liem SE, Asad S, Read SE, Joshi S. Resistance to human immunodeficiency virus type 1 (HIV-1) infection in human CD4+ lymphocyte-derived cell lines conferred by using retroviral vectors expressing an HIV-1 RNA-specific ribozyme. J Virol 1991; 65:5531-5534.

68. Leavitt MC, Yu M, Yamada O et al. Transfer of an anti-HIV-1 ribozyme gene into primary human lymphocytes. Human Gene Therapy 1994; 5:1115-1120.

69. Yu M, Leavitt MC, Maruyama M et al. Intracellular immunization of human fetal cord blood stem/progenitor cells with a ribozyme against human immunodeficiency virus type 1. Proc Natl Acad Sci USA 1995; 92:669-703.

70. Trono D, Feinberg MB, Baltimore D. HIV-gag mutants can dominantly interfere with the replication of the wild-type virus. Cell 1989; 59:113-120.

71. Sczakiel G, Pawlita M, Kleinheinz A. Specific inhibition of human immunodeficiency virus type 1 replication by RNA transcribed in sense and antisense from the 5'-leader/gag region. Biochem Biophys Res Comm 1990; 169:643-651.

72. Sczakiel G, Pawlita M. Inhibition of human immunodeficiency virus type 1 replication in human T cells stably expressing antisense RNA. J Virol 1991; 65:468-472.

73. Veres G, Escaich S, Baker J et al. Intracellular expression of RNA transcripts complementary to the human immunodeficiency virus type 1 *gag* gene inhibits viral replication in human CD4+ lymphocytes. J Virol 1996; 70:8792-8800.

74. Sarver N, Cantin EM, Chang PS et al. Ribozymes as potential anti-HIV-1 therapeutic agents. Science 1990; 247:1222-1225.

75. Rice WG, Supko JG, Malspeis L et al. Inhibitors of HIV nucleoprotein Zinc fingers as candidates for the treatment of AIDS. Science 1995; 270:1194-1197.

76. Mebatsion T, Finke S, Weiland F, Conzelman K-K. A CXCR4/CD4 pseudotype rhabdovirus that selectively infects HIV-1 envelope protein-expressing cells. Cell 1997; 90:841-847.

77. Schnell MJ, Johnson JE, Buonocore L, Rose JK. Construction of a novel virus that targets HIV-1-infected cells and controls HIV-1 infection. Cell 1997; 90:849-857.

78. Marasco WA, Haseltine WA, Chen S. Design, intracellular expression, and activity of a human anti-human immunodeficiency virus type 1 gp120 single-chain antibody. Proc Natl Acad Sci USA 1993; 90:7889-7893.

79. Chen C-J, Banerjea AC, Harmison GG, Haglund K, Schubert M. Multitarget-ribozyme directed to cleave at up to nine highly conserved HIV-1 env RNA regions inhibits HIV-1 replication—potential effectiveness against most presently sequenced HIV-1 isolates. Nucleic Acids Res 1992; 20:4581-4589.

80. Babé LM, Rosé J, Craik CS. Trans-dominant inhibitory immunodeficiency virus type 1 protease monomers prevent protease activation and virion maturation. Proc Natl Acad Sci USA 1995; 92: 10069-10073.

81. Junker U, Escaich S, Plavec I et al. Intracellular expression of human immunodeficiency virus type 1 (HIV-1) protease variants inhibits replication of wild-type and protease inhibitor-resistant HIV-1 strains in human T cell lines. J Virol 1996; 70:7765-7772.

82. Serio D, Rizvi TA, Cartas M et al. Development of a novel anti-HIV-1 agent from within: Effect of chimeric vpr-containing protease cleavage site residues on virus replication. Proc Natl Acad Sci USA 1997; 94:3346-3351.

83. Trono D. HIV accessory proteins: leading roles for the supporting cast. Cell 1995; 82:189-192.

84. Miller RH, Turk SR, Black RJ, Bridges S, Sarver N. Conference summary: Novel HIV therapies—from discovery to clinical proof of concept. AIDS Res Hum Retroviruses 1996; 12:859-865.

85. Heinzinger NK, Bukrinsky MI, Haggerty SA et al. The Vpr protein of human immunodeficiency virus type 1 influences nuclear localization of viral nucleic acids in nondividing host cells. Proc Natl Acad Sci USA 1994; 91:7311-7315.

86. Miller RH, Sarver N. HIV accessory proteins as therapeutic targets. Nature Med 1997; 4:389-394.

87. Wu X, Liu H, Xiao H et al. Targeting foreign proteins to human immunodeficiency virus particles via fusion with vpr and vpx. J Virol 1995; 69:3389-3398.

88. Lever A, Gottlinger H, Haseltine W, Sodroski J. Identification of a sequence required for efficient packaging of human immunodeficiency virus type 1 RNA into virions. J Virol 1989; 63:4085-4087.

89. Mann R, Baltimore D. Varying the position of a retrovirus packaging sequence results in the encapsidation of both unspliced and spliced RNAs. J Virol 1985; 54:401-407.

90. Sun L-Q, Warrilow D, Wang L, Witherington C, Macpherson J, Symonds G. Ribozyme-mediated suppression of Moloney murine leukemia virus and human immunodeficiency virus type 1 replication in permissive cell lines. Proc Natl Acad Sci USA 1994; 91:9715-9719.

91. Caruso M, Klatzmann D. Selective killing of CD4+ cells harboring a human immunodeficiency virus-inducible suicide gene prevents viral spread in an infected population. Proc Natl Acad Sci USA 1992; 89:182-186.

92. Brady HJM, Miles CG, Pennington DJ, Dzierzak EA. Specific ablation of human immunodeficiency virus Tat-expressing cells by conditionally toxic retroviruses. Proc Natl Acad Sci USA 1994; 91:356-369.

93. Venkatesh LK, Arens MQ, Subramanian T, Chinnadurai G. Selective inhibition of toxicity to human cells expressing human immunodeficiency virus type 1 Tat by a conditionally cytotoxic adenovirus vector. Proc Natl Acad Sci USA 1990; 87:8746-8750.

94. Harrison GS, Long CJ, Curiel TJ, Maxwell F, Maxwell IH. Inhibition of human immunodeficiency virus-1 production resulting from transduction with a retrovirus containing an HIV-regulated diphteria toxin A chain gene. Human Gene Ther 1992; 3:461-469.

95. Harrison GS, Long CJ, Maxwell F, Glode LM, Maxwell IH. Inhibition of HIV production in cells containing an integrated, HIV-regulated diptheria toxin A chain gene. AIDS Res Hum Retroviruses 1992.

96. Winters MA, Merigan TC. Continuous presence of CD4-PE40 is required for antiviral activity against single-passage HIV isolates and infected peripheral blood mononuclear cells. AIDS Res Hum Retroviruses 1993; 9:1091-1096.

97. Hamouda T, McPhee R, Hsia S-C, Read S, Holland TC, King SR. Inhibition of human immunodeficiency virus replication by the herpes simplex virus virion host shutoff protein. J Virol 1997; 71:5521-5527.

98. Dalgleish AG, Beverley PCL, Clapham PR, Crawford DH, Greaves MF, Weiss RA. The CD4 (T4) antigen is an essential component of the receptor for the AIDS retrovirus. Nature 1984; 312:763-767.

99. Daar ES, Li XL, Moudgil T, Ho DD. High concentrations of recombinant soluble CD4 are required to neutralize primary Human Immunodeficiency Virus Type 1 isolates. Proc Natl Acad Sci USA 1990; 87:6574-6578.

100. Watanabe M, Chen ZW, Tsubota H, Lord CI, Levine CG, Letvin NL. Soluble human CD4 elicits antibody responses in rhesus monkeys that inhibits simian immunodeficiency virus replication. Proc Natl Acad Sci USA 1991; 88:120-124.

101. Watanabe M, Boyson JE, Lord CI, Letvin NL. Chimpanzees immunized with recombinant soluble CD4 develop anti-self CD4 antibody responses with anti-human immunodeficiency virus activity. Proc Natl Acad Sci USA 1992; 89:5103-5107.

102. Buonocore L, Rose JK. Prevention of HIV-1 glycoprotein transport by soluble CD4 retained in the endoplasmic reticulum. Nature 1990; 345:625-628.

103. Buoncore L, Rose JK. Blockade of human immunodeficiency virus type 1 production in CD4+ T cells by an intracellular CD4 expressed under control of the viral long terminal repeat. Proc Natl Acad Sci USA 1993; 90:2695-2699.

104. Alkhatib G, Combardiere C, Broder CC et al. CC CKR5: A RANTES, MIP-1α, MIP-1β receptor as a fusion cofactor for macrophage-tropic HIV-1. Science 1996; 272:1955-1958.

105. Choe H, Farzan M, Sun Y et al. The β-Chemokine receptors CCR3 and CCR5 facilitate infection by primary HIV-1 isolates. Cell 1996; 85:1135-1148.

106. Deng H, Liu R, Ellmeier W et al. Identification of a major coreceptor for primary isolates of HIV-1. Nature 1996; 381:661-666.

107. Doranz BJ, Rucker J, Yi Y et al. A dual-tropic primary HIV-1 isolate that uses Fusin and the β-Chemokine receptors CKR-5, CKR-3, and CKR-2b as Fusion cofactors. Cell 1996; 85:1149-1158.

108. Dragic T, Litwin V, Allaway GP et al. HIV-1 entry into CD4+ cells is mediated by the chemokine receptor CC-CKR-5. Nature 1996; 381:667-673.

109. Feng Y, Broder CC, Kennedy PE, Berger EA. HIV-1 entry cofactor: functional cDNA cloning of a seven-transmembrane, G protein-coupled receptor. Science 1996; 272:872-877.

110. Baggiolini M, Dewald B, Moser B. Interleukin-8 and related chemotactic cytokines-CXC and CC chemokines. Adv Immunol 1994; 55:97-179.

111. Cocchi F, DeVico AL, Garzino-Demo A, Arya SK, Gallo RC, Lusso P. Indentification of RANTES, MIP1α, and MIP-1β as the major HIV-suppressive factors produced by CD8+ T cells. Science 1995; 270:1811-1815.

112. Paxton WA, Martin SR, Tse D et al. Relative resistance to HIV-1 infection of CD4 lymphocytes from persons who remain uninfected despite multiple high-risk sexual exposures. Nature Med 1996; 2:412-417.

113. Liu R, Paxton WA, Choe S et al. Homozygous defect in HIV-1 coreceptor accounts for resistance of some multiply-exposed individuals to HIV-1 infection. Cell 1996; 86:367-377.

114. Dean M, Carrington M, Winkler C et al. Genetic restriction of HIV-1 infection and progression to AIDS by a deletion allele of the *CKR5* structural gene. Science 1996; 273:1856-1862.

115. Yang AG, Bai X, Huang XF, Yao C, Chen S. Phenotypic knockout of HIV type 1 chemokine coreceptor CCR-5 by intrakines as potential therapeutic approach for HIV-1 infection. Proc Natl Acad Sci USA 1997; 94:11567-11572.

116. Nabel G, Baltimore D. An inducible transcription factor activates expression of human immunodeficiency virus in T cells. Nature 1987; 326:711-713.

117. Baeuerle PA, Baltimore D. IκB: a specific inhibitor of the NF-κB transcription factor. Science 1988; 242:540-546.

118. Urban MB, Baeuerle PA. The 65-kD subunit of NF-κB is a receptor for IkB and a modulator of DNA-binding specificity. Genes Dev 1990; 4:1975-1984.

119. Laspia MF, Rice AP, Mathews MB. Synergy between HIV-1 Tat and adenovirus E1A is principally due to stabilization of transcriptional elongation. Genes Dev 1990; 4:2397-2408.

120. Wu BY, Wofferdin C, Duckett CS, Ohno T, Nabel GJ. Regulation of human retoviral latency by the NF-κB/IκB family: inhibition of human immunodeficiency virus replication by IκB through a rev-dependent mechanism. Proc. Natl. Acad. Sci. USA 1995; 92:1480-1484.

121. Beauparlant P, Kwon H, Clarke M et al. Transdominant mutants of IκB block Tat-tumor necrosis factor synergistic activation of human immunodeficiency virus type 1 gene expression and virus multiplication. J Virol 1996; 70:5777-5785.

122. Ruhl M, Himmelspach M, Bahr GM et al. Eukaryotic initiation factor 5A is a cellular target of the human immunodeficiency virus type 1 Rev activation domain mediating trans-activation. J Cell Biol 1993; 123:1309-1320.

123. Bevec D, Jaksche H, Oft M et al. Inhibition of HIV-1 replication in lymphocytes by mutants of the Rev cofactor eIF-5A. Science 1996; 271:1858-1860.

124. Junker U, Bevec D, Barske C et al. Intracellular expression of cellular eIF-5A mutants inhibits HIV-1 replication in human T cells: a feasibility study. Human Gene Ther 1996; 7:1861-1869.

125. Francis ML, Meltzer MS, Gendelman HE. Interferons in the persistence, pathogenesis, and treatment of HIV infection. AIDS Res Hum Retroviruses 1992; 8:199-207.

126. Baca-Regen L, Heinzinger N, Stevenson M, Gendelman HE. Alpha interferon-induced antiretroviral activites: restriction of viral nucleic acid synthesis and progeny virion production in human immunodeficiency virus type 1-infected monocytes. J Virol 1994; 68:7559-7565.

127. Constantoulakis P, Campbell M, Felber BK, Nasioulas G, Afonina E, Pavlakis GN. Inhibition of Rev-mediated HIV-1 expression by an RNA binding protein encoded by the Interferon-inducible 9-27 gene. Science 1993; 259:1314-1318.

128. Vieillard V, Lauret E, Rousseau V, De Maeyer E. Blocking of retroviral infection at a step prior to reverse transcription in cells transformed to constitutively express interferon beta. Proc Natl Acad Sci USA 1994; 91:2689-2693.

129. Vieillard V, Lauret E, Maguer V et al. Autocrine interferon-β synthesis for gene therapy of HIV infection: increased resistance to HIV-1 in lymphocytes from healthy and HIV-infected individuals. AIDS 1995; 9:1221-1228.

130. Schnittman SM, Vogel S, Baseler M, Lane HC, Davey RT. A phase I study of interferon-alpha 2b in combination with interleukin-2 in patients with Human Immunodeficiency Virus infection. J Infect Dis 1994; 169:981-989.

131. Perkins ND, Agranoff AB, Duckett CS, Nabel GJ. Transcription factor AP-2 regulates Human Immunodeficiency Virus Type 1 gene expression. J Virol 1994; 68:6820-6823.

132. Jones KA, Kadonaga JT, Luciw PA, Tjian R. Activation of the AIDS retrovirus promoter by the cellular transcription factor, Sp1. Science 1986; 232:755-759.

133. Perkins ND, Agranoff AB, Pascal E, Nabel GJ. An interaction between the DNA-binding domains of RelA(p65) and Sp1 mediates human immunodeficiency virus gene activation. Mol Cell Biol 1994; 14:6570-6583.

134. Stade K, Ford CS, Guthrie C, Weis K. Exportin 1 (Crm1p) is an essential nuclear export factor. Cell 1997; 90:1041-1050.

135. Fornerod M, Ohno M, Yoshida M, Mattaj IW. CRM1 is an export receptor for leucine-rich nuclear export signals. Cell 1997; 90:1051-1060.

136. Ullman KS, Powers MA, Forbes DJ. Nuclear export receptors: From importin to exportin. Cell 1997; 90:967-970.

137. Bogerd HP, Fridell RA, Madore S, Cullen BR. Identification of a novel cellular cofactor for the rev/rex class of retroviral regulatory proteins. Cell 1995; 82:485-494.

138. Powell DM, Amaral MC, Wu JY, Maniatis T, Greene WC. HIV Rev-dependent binding of SF2/ASF to the Rev response element: possible role in Rev-mediated inhibition of HIV RNA splicing. Proc Natl Acad Sci USA 1997; 94:973-978.

139. Yuyama N, Ohkawa J, Koguma T, Shirai M, Taira K. A multifunctional expression vector for an anti-HIV-1 ribozyme that produces a 5'- and 3'-trimmed trans-acting ribozyme, targeted against HIV-1 RNA, and cis-acting ribozymes that are designed to bind to and thereby sequester trans-activator proteins such as Tat and Rev. Nucleic Acids Res 1994; 22:5060-5067.

140. Yamada O, Kraus G, Luznik L, Yu M, Wong-Staal F. A chimeric human immunodeficiency virus type 1 (HIV-1) minimal rev response element-ribozyme molecule exhibits dual antiviral function and inhibits cell-cell transmission of HIV-1. J Virol 1996; 70:1596-1601.

141. Ulich C, Harrich D, Estes P, Gaynor RB. Inhibition of human immunodeficiency virus Type 1 replication is enhanced by a combination of transdominant tat and rev proteins. J Virol 1996; 70:4871-4876.

142. Ohkawa J, Yuyama N, Takebe Y, Nishikawa S, Taira K. Importance of independence in ribozyme reactions: kinetic behavior of trimmed and simply connected ribozymes with potential activity against human immunodeficiency virus. Proc Natl Acad Sci USA 1993; 90:11302-11306.

143. Kinter AL, Bende SM, Hardy EC, Jackson R, Fauci AS. Interleukin 2 induces CD8+ T cell-mediated suppression of human immunodeficiency virus replication in CD4+ T cells and this effect overrides its ability to stimulate virus expression. Proc Natl Acad Sci USA 1995; 92:10985-10989.

144. Barker E, Mackewicz CE, Levy JA. Effects of TH1 and TH2 cytokines on CD8+ cell response against human immunodeficiency virus: Implications for long-term survival. Proc Natl Acad Sci USA 1995; 92:11135-11139.

145. Carmichael A, Jin X, Sissons P, Borysiewicz. Quantitative analysis of the human immunodeficiency virus type 1 (HIV-1)-specific cytotoxic T lymphocyte (CTL) response at different stages of HIV-1 infection: differential CTL responses to HIV-1 and Epstein-Barr Virus in late disease. J Exp Med 1993; 177:249-256.

146. Kundu SK, Merigan TC. Inverse relationship of CD8+CD11+ suppressor T cells with human immunodeficiency virus (HIV)-specific cellular cytotoxicity and natural killer cell activity in HIV infection. Immunology 1991; 74:567-571.

147. Koup RA, Safrit JT, Cao Y et al. Temporal association of cellular immune responses with the initial control of viremia in primary human immunodeficiency virus type 1 syndrome. J Virol 1994; 68:4650-4655.
148. Klein MR, van Baalen CA, Holwerda AM et al. Kinetics of gag-specific cytotoxic T lymphocyte responses during the clinical course of HIV-1 infection: a longitudinal analysis of rapid progressors and long-term asymptomatics. J Exp Med 1995; 181:1365-1372.
149. Borrow P, Lewicki H, Hahn BH, Shaw GM, Oldstone MBA. Virus-specific CD8+ cytotoxic T lymphocyte activity associated with control of viremia in primary human immunodeficiency virus type 1 infection. J Virol 1994; 68:6103-6110.
150. Blaese RM. Steps toward gene therapy: 2. Cancer and AIDS. Hosp Pract 1995; 30:37-45.
151. Flowers CC, Wofferdin C, Petryniak J, Yang S, Nabel GJ. Inhibition of recombinant human immunodeficiency virus type 1 replication by a site-specific recombinase. J Virol 1997; 71:2685-2692.
152. Riddell SR, Elliott M, Lewinsohn DA et al. T cell mediated rejection of gene-modified HIV-specific cytotoxic T lymphocytes in HIV-infected patients. Nature Med 1996; 2:216-223.
153. Ziegner UHM, Peters G, Jolly DJ et al. Cytotoxic T lymphocyte induction in asymptomatic HIV-1-infected patients immunized with Retrovector®-transduced autologous fibroblasts expressing HIV-1 IIIB env/rev proteins. AIDS 1995; 9:43-50.
154. Ross G, Erickson R, Knorr D et al. Gene therapy in the United States: A five year status report. Hum Gene Ther 1996; 7:1781-1790.
155. Baltimore D. The enigma of HIV infection. Cell 1995; 82:175-176.

CHAPTER 3

Trans-Splicing Ribozymes as Potential HIV Gene Inhibitors

Seong-Wook Lee and Bruce A. Sullenger

Introduction

The observation that certain ribozymes can perform trans-splicing reactions has engendered much speculation about the potential utility of such RNA catalysts as anti-HIV agents. Here we will provide an example of how this trans-splicing reaction can be employed to revise HIV transcripts to give them antiviral activity. Then we will quickly review the splicing reaction mediated by the group I ribozyme from *Tetrahymena thermophila* and highlight some of the facets of this reaction which make it potentially amenable to gene therapy applications.

Ribozymes as Potential Anti-HIV Agents

Certain RNA molecules can adopt three-dimensional conformations which allow them to perform enzymatic reactions. These RNA enzymes or ribozymes contain catalytic cores and active sites which allow them to catalyze cleavage and ligation reactions upon specific substrate RNAs with rate enhancements similar to those achieved by many protein enzymes. A hammerhead ribozyme is a small cis-cleaving ribozyme motif which was isolated from the self-cleaving satellite RNA of tobacco ringspot virus. An enzymatic version of this ribozyme has been created by in vitro mutagenesis which is capable of cleaving novel substrate RNAs in test tubes with multiple turnover.[1] This relatively small RNA enzyme (approximately 36 nucleotides in length) has been extensively studied by in vitro biochemical techniques. It contains a guide sequence which allows

Gene Therapy for HIV Infection, edited by Clay Smith. © 1998 Springer-Verlag and R.G. Landes Company.

it to base pair with and subsequently cleave specific substrate RNAs present in trans. Specific substrate sequence requirements are minimal, allowing for the design of a particular ribozyme capable of cleaving a designated RNA by adjusting the length and composition of the ribozyme's guide sequence. Its small size and malleability makes this ribozyme a very attractive potential gene inhibitor.[2,3] Virtually any transcript including those encoding HIV early genes products can be targeted for cleavage and subsequent destruction (Fig. 3.1). In fact, several groups have demonstrated that such trans-cleaving ribozymes can be exploited to inhibit HIV replication in immortalized human cells including CD4+ T cells when such cells are challenged with a moderately-low inoculum of virus.[2,4]

Limitations of Trans-Cleaving Ribozymes as HIV Inhibitors

Several potential problems exist for the application of trans-cleaving ribozymes to HIV inhibition. First, HIV RNAs can easily mutate to avoid being cleaved by ribozymes. A point mutation at the ribozyme cleavage site should abolish ribozyme-mediated cleavage and destruction of viral transcripts. To address this concern, researchers have intentionally targeted highly conserved regions in the viral RNA for cleavage. In addition, most researchers have proposed generating a number of ribozymes directed against a variety of target sites on the HIV viral transcripts so that multiple mutations will be required for the virus to escape the ribozyme-mediated inhibition.

Second, trans-cleaving ribozyme reaction products are not stable inside mammalian cells.[3] Thus it has been almost impossible to systematically determine what influences RNA catalysis inside mammalian cells using such cleaving ribozymes. Therefore, no rational approach to improving the effectiveness and safety of cleaving ribozymes has been developed.

Finally, trans-cleaving ribozymes will have to cut virtually 100% of the HIV RNAs in an infected cell to effectively stop viral replication. This level of efficiency may be very difficult to achieve in practice especially when trying to inhibit highly expressed genes such as viral ones. For example, in a recent tissue culture study using a hammerhead ribozyme, substrate expression was reduced by 90%, but further reduction was extremely difficult to achieve.[3]

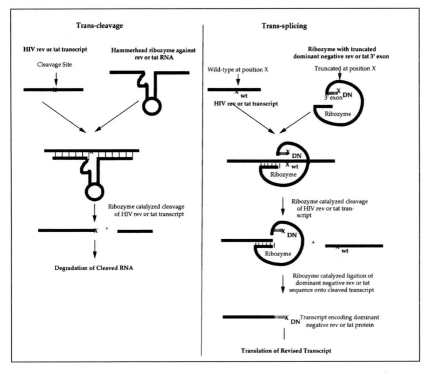

Fig. 3.1. Ribozyme mediated trans-cleavage vs. trans-splicing to inhibit HIV replication. DN=dominant negative sequence, wt=wild type sequence.

Advantages of Trans-Splicing Ribozymes

In contrast to the trans-cleaving ribozymes (such as the hammerhead and hairpin ribozymes), the group I and group II splicing ribozymes naturally perform both cleavage and ligation reactions.[5] Recently, such splicing reactions have been employed to modify targeted transcripts inside cells.[6,7] Using these splicing ribozymes, one can directly evaluate ribozyme reactions that occur in vivo to generate ribozyme constructs that will not simply destroy HIV transcripts but rather alter them to make them encode anti-HIV agents. In other words, through the use of trans-splicing ribozymes, one can alter HIV RNAs and turn them against the virus (Fig. 3.1). This approach should simultaneously reduce the concentration of functional viral proteins present in an infected cell and engender the production of anti-viral proteins. Moreover, in contrast to inhibition strategies that express dominant negative versions of HIV proteins such as RevM10 as described in chapter 2, anti-viral protein production engendered by trans-splicing should not elicit an immune response to transduced cells that are not infected by HIV, because inhibitory proteins can only be produced in cells expressing the viral RNA target transcripts.[8,9] Furthermore, in contrast to cleavage of HIV RNAs, ribozyme-mediated revision of HIV transcripts will probably not require a 100 percent reaction efficiency to inhibit viral replication (Fig. 3.1). Rather, we expect that if a trans-splicing ribozyme changes only a fraction of the viral transcripts to ones encoding dominant mutant versions of the rev or tat protein, then the ribozyme will effectively inhibit HIV replication. In addition, because the trans-splicing ribozymes generate reaction products that are stable in cells and trans-cleaving ribozymes do not, it will be much easier to study and optimize trans-splicing reactions.[3,6,7,10] For these reasons, trans-splicing ribozymes represent potentially powerful reagents for therapeutic applications, including their use for the inhibition of HIV replication.

Targeted Trans-Splicing by the *Tetrahymena* Ribozyme

RNA Revision By Ribozymes

During gene expression, the information contained in a given protein encoding gene is directly copied into the corresponding premessenger RNA by transcription. The information embedded in this RNA is not fixed, however, and can be modified by splicing or editing to remove, add or rewrite parts of the initial transcript.[11-17] The self-splicing reaction catalyzed by the group I intron ribozyme from *Tetrahymena thermophila* is perhaps the most thoroughly understood reaction that revises RNA. The intron performs two consecutive trans-esterification reactions to liberate itself and join flanking exons (Fig. 3.2A).[18] In the first, an intron bound guanosine attacks the phosphodiester bond at the 5' splice site that is defined by a conserved G-U base pair. In the second, the free 3' hydroxyl group, now present on the end of the cleaved 5' exon, attacks the phosphorus atom at the 3' splice site to result in the liberation of the intron and the ligation of the 5' and 3' exons. Careful characterization of this reaction over the past decade has illustrated that the vast majority of sequence requirements for this self-splicing are contained within the intron. No specific sequence requirements exist for the 3' exon in this reaction, and the only specific sequence requirement for 5' exons is to have a uridine (U) preceding the cleavage site.[5,18] In addition, base pairing must be maintained between the end of the 5' exon and the 5' exon-binding site on the ribozyme so that the ribozyme can hold onto the 5' exon after cleavage. These base pairs can be composed of any set of complementary nucleotides, however.

Ribozyme Mediated Trans-Splicing

In addition to performing a self-splicing reaction, a slightly shortened version of the group I ribozyme from *Tetrahymena* (called the L-21 form) can splice an exon attached to its 3' end onto a targeted 5' exon RNA that is present in trans (Fig. 3.2B). In this reaction, the 5' exon is recognized by the group I ribozyme via base pairing through its 5' exon binding site. In the process of pairing, a U is positioned across from the guanosine present at the 5' end of the 5' exon binding site. Once positioned, the ribozyme catalyzes the cleavage of the substrate RNA at the reconstructed 5' splice site and then ligates its 3' exon onto the 5' exon cleavage product (Fig. 3.2B). Trans-splicing by group I ribozymes is extremely malleable because, as mentioned above, very few sequence requirements exist for the exons in this reaction. Virtually any U residue in a 5' exon can be targeted for splicing by altering the nucleotide composition of the 5' exon binding site on the ribozyme to make it complementary to the target site. Because no specific 3' exon sequences are required, such trans-splicing ribozymes can potentially be employed to splice virtually any 3' exon sequence onto a targeted U residue. Thus, such trans-splicing reactions can in principle be employed to rewrite genetic instructions for a variety of applications, including the repair of mutant transcripts and the revision of pathogenic RNAs.

To assess the feasibility of this approach, a simple model system has been developed in which a truncated *lacZ* transcript is repaired through targeted trans-splicing (Fig. 3.3). A ribozyme was generated that could recognize the truncated *lacZ* RNA via base-pairing, cleave it, release additional residues, and subsequently splice onto the trimmed 5' exon a 3' exon carried in by the ribozyme that encodes the next 200 nucleotides of *lacZ*. The process should result in the production of a repaired transcript which contains the entire coding sequence for the translation of the alpha complement of β-galactosidase. As reported, this RNA repair reaction can proceed fairly quickly and with an 85% efficiency under pseudo-physiological conditions in a test tube.[6]

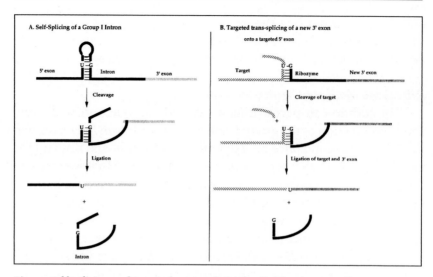

Fig. 3.2. Self-splicing and targeted trans-splicing by the *Tetrahymena* ribozyme.

Targeted Trans-Splicing in Escherichia Coli

To determine if similar reactions could proceed inside of cells, both the ribozyme-3' *lacZ*-exon RNA and the truncated 5' *lacZ*-exon RNA were expressed from T7 RNA polymerase promoters in *E. coli*.[6] Total RNA was isolated from cells expressing the ribozyme and the mutant *lacZ* transcript and analyzed for the presence of repaired *lacZ* RNAs. Reverse transcription-PCR (RT/PCR) analysis was performed with one primer specific for the 5' exon and the other specific for the 3' exon sequences of *lacZ*. Therefore, amplified fragments should only be generated if the repaired RNA were present in the sample. Repaired transcripts were detected only in RNAs from cells which contained an active ribozyme and T7 RNA polymerase. From this analysis, it was concluded that trans-splicing could occur in *E. coli*. In addition, sequence analysis of the amplified products demonstrated that the ribozyme was faithfully correcting the truncated transcript and in the process restoring the open reading frame for the translation of the alpha complement of β-galactosidase. To determine if these repaired transcripts were being translated in *E. coli*, a simple colorimetric assay was performed to test for β-galactosidase activity. This analysis demonstrated that the repaired transcripts were being translated. In summary, the *Tetrahymena* group I ribozyme can correctly repair mutant *lacZ* transcripts in *E. coli* by targeted trans-splicing.[6]

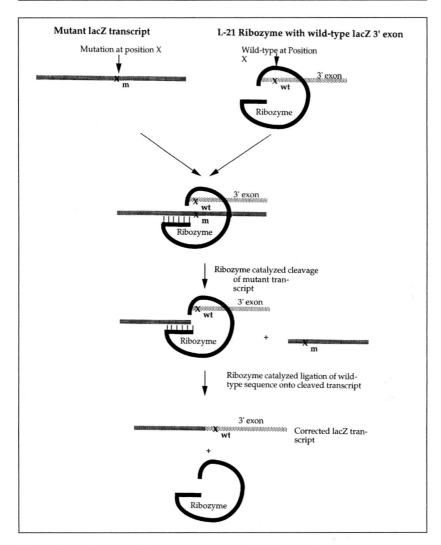

Fig. 3.3. Targeted trans-splicing to correct mutant lacZ transcripts.

Targeted Trans-Splicing in Mammalian Cells

To determine if such trans-splicing could proceed in a more therapeutically relevant setting, the ribozyme-3' *lacZ*-exon RNA and the truncated 5' *lacZ*-exon RNA were expressed from T7 RNA polymerase promoters in a mouse fibroblast cell line called OST7-1 that contains T7 RNA polymerase.[19] For trans-splicing to occur, the ribozyme must recognize the targeted *lacZ* substrate RNA via base pairing, cleave it, release the downstream product and attach its restorative *lacZ*-3' exon (Fig. 3.3). To monitor targeted trans-splicing in transfected OST7-1 cells, total RNA was isolated and reaction products were amplified by reverse transcription and the polymerase chain reaction (RT/PCR). RT/PCR was performed using one primer specific for the targeted 5' *lacZ* sequence and the other primer specific for the restorative *lacZ* 3' exon. An amplified fragment of expected size (200 base pairs) was generated from RNA isolated from the OST7-1 cells transfected with a plasmid that encodes for the active ribozyme and the *lacZ* target RNA. In contrast, no such amplified product was generated from RNA from mock transfected cells or from cells transfected with the inactive ribozyme containing plasmid. From these results, it was concluded that a group I ribozyme can trans-splice its 3' exon onto targeted transcripts in mammalian cells and that this 3' exon provides a convenient molecular tag that allows one to directly follow RNA catalysis in a therapeutically relevant setting for the first time. This analysis provides direct evidence that the ribozyme reaction proceeds as anticipated in mammalian cells and suggests that adequately developed RNA repair of deleterious mutant transcripts or revision of pathogenic transcripts in human cells may be a viable approach to human gene therapy.[20,21]

Conclusions

Trans-splicing ribozymes can be employed to rewrite genetic instructions. Thus they can potentially be employed to revise HIV RNAs to give them anti-viral activity. The potential utility of this approach for blocking HIV replication has yet to be tested. Several parameters of the splicing reaction will, however, likely have to be optimized before this approach is useful. The efficiency of the splicing reaction will likely have to be moderately high. Recently it has been demonstrated that a trans-splicing ribozyme can react with up to 50% of a specific target RNA in mammalian cells.[10] If this level of efficiency can be obtained in the case of revising HIV messages, then the trans-splicing approach may prove to be able to substantially inhibit HIV replication. Even if this level of efficiency can be obtained, other hurdles (such as efficient gene transfer into the appropriate cells) will have to be overcome for the trans-splicing approach to HIV gene therapy to be useful in the clinic. In this regard, this approach shares many of the same challenges faced by other HIV gene therapy strategies.

References

1. Hasseloff J, Gerlach W. Simple RNA enzymes with new and highly specific endoribonuclease activities. Nature 1988; 334:585-589.
2. Sarver N, Cantin E et al. Ribozymes as potential anti-HIV-1 therapeutic agents. Science 1990; 247:1222-1225.
3. Sullenger BA, Cech TR. Tethering ribozymes to a retroviral packaging signal for destruction of viral RNA. Science 1993; 262:1566-1569.
4. Yu M, Ojwang J et al. A hairpin ribozyme inhibits expression of diverse strains of human immunodeficiency virus type 1. Proc Natl Acad Sci USA 1993; 90:6340-6344.
5. Cech TR. Structure and mechanism of the large catalytic RNAs: Group I and group II introns and ribonuclease P. In: Gestsland RF, Atkins JF eds. The RNA World. New York: Cold Spring Harbor Laboratory Press, 1993:239-269.
6. Sullenger BA, Cech TR. Ribozyme-mediated repair of defective mRNA by targeted trans-splicing. Nature 1994; 317:619-622.
7. Jones JT, Lee S-W, Sullenger BA. Tagging ribozyme reaction sites to follow trans-splicing in mammalian cells. Nature Medicine 1996; 2:643-648.
8. Malim M, Bohnlein E, Hauber J et al. Functional dissection of the HIV rev transactivator-derivation of a transdominant repressor of rev function. Cell 1989; 58:205-214.
9. Malim M, Freimuth W et al. Stable expression of transdominant rev protein in human T cells inhibits human immunodeficiency virus replication. J Exp Med 1992; 176:1197-1201.
10. Jones JT, Sullenger BA. Evaluating and enhancing ribozyme reaction efficiency in mammalian cells. Nature Biotechnology 1997; 15:902-905.
11. Moore MJ, Query CC, Sharp PA. Splicing of precursors to mRNAs by the spliceosome. In: Gestsland RF, Atkins JF eds. The RNA World. New York: Cold Spring Harbor Laboratory Press, 1993:303-357.
12. Ruby SW, Abelson J. Pre-mRNA splicing in yeast. Trends Genet 1991; 7:79-85.
13. Guthrie C. Messenger RNA splicing in yeast: clues to why the spliceosome is a ribonucleoprotein. Science 1991; 253:157-163.
14. Green MR. Biochemical mechanisms of constitutive and regulated pre-mRNA splicing. Annu Rev Cell Biol 1991; 7:559-599.
15. Bass BL. RNA editing: new uses for old players in the RNA world. In: Gestsland RF, Atkins JF eds. The RNA World. New York: Cold Spring Harbor Laboratory Press, 1993:383-418.
16. Benne RJ, Tromp MC. Major transcript of the frameshifted *coxII* gene from trypanosome mitochondria contains four nucleotides that are not encoded in the DNA. Cell 1986; 46:819-826.
17. Sollner-Webb B. RNA editing. Curr Opin Cell Biol 1991; 3:1056-1061.
18. Cech TR. Self-splicing of group I introns. Ann Rev Biochem 1990; 59:543-568.

19. Elroy-Stein O, Moss B. Cytoplasmic expression system based upon constitutive synthesis of bacteriophage T7 RNA polymerase in mammalian cells. Proc Natl Acad Sci USA 1990; 81:6743-6747.

20. Sullenger BA, Cech TR. RNA repair: a new possibility for gene therapy. Journal of NIH Research 1995; 7:46-47.

21. Sullenger BA. Revising messages traveling along the cellular information superhighway. Chemistry & Biology 1995; 2:249-253.

CHAPTER 4

Viral Vectors for HIV Gene Therapy

Kenneth L. Phillips

Introduction

The goal of gene therapy for the treatment of acquired immuno deficiency syndrome (AIDS) is suppression of human immunodeficiency virus (HIV) replication at any stage of the viral life cycle in order to promote host survival. As described in chapter 2, most current gene therapy efforts focus on:

1. postexposure vaccination; or
2. expression of anti-HIV-1 genes in cells permissive for HIV infection, i.e., "intracellular immunization".[1]

Intracellular immunization strategies include both RNA-based (ribozymes, RNA decoys, anti-sense RNA) and protein-based (transdominant viral proteins, intracellular antibodies) gene based inhibitors. All of these approaches have been shown to block HIV replication in cell culture model systems. However, the inefficiency of currently available gene delivery systems may limit their clinical application. Therapeutic genes must be efficiently transferred and maintained in targeted hematopoietic cells to be of therapeutic value.

To date, recombinant animal viruses provide the most efficient means for achieving heterologous gene transfer and expression in mammalian cells.[2] Viral vectors which integrate into the host genome of targeted cells provide stable gene transfer and expression.[2] In contrast, viruses which fail to integrate and replicate as episomes, e.g., adenovirus, are limited for HIV gene therapy because infection and transgene expression do not persist.[2] These vectors also elicit an immune response in the host which contributes to their

Gene Therapy for HIV Infection, edited by Clay Smith. © 1998 Springer-Verlag and R.G. Landes Company.

instability.[2] Therefore, the most promising gene transfer modalities for HIV gene therapy are based upon integrating retroviral and adeno-associated virus (AAV) vectors. The aim of this review is to summarize the current understanding and progress in retrovirus and AAV based gene transfer technology for HIV gene therapy.

Retrovirus Gene Transfer Systems

Taxonomy

The Retroviridae are single stranded enveloped RNA viruses which have historically been classified on the basis of virion morphology and pathogenic potential.[3] The Oncoviridae subgroup are well known for inducing neoplasia in the host and include the well characterized murine leukemia viruses (MLV) and human T cell leukemia virus type 1 and 2 (HTLV-I and -II).[3] The Spumaviridae subgroup, including the human foamy virus (HFV), have not yet been associated with any disease but induce a 'foamy' cytopathic effect in infected host cells.[3] The Lentiviridae subgroup include the human immunodeficiency viruses type 1 and 2 (HIV-1 and -2) and are well known for inducing chronic disease with an indirect role in neoplasia.[3]

Retrovirus Life Cycle

The retroviral life cycle initiates with binding of the viral envelope glycoprotein to a specific cell surface receptor on the host cell membrane(Fig. 4.1).[3] Several receptors are cloned and characterized, and most retroviruses utilize a single receptor for entry.[4] In contrast, HIV utilizes both CD4 and cell specific coreceptors termed Fusin and chemokine receptor 5 (CC-CKR-5).[4] Amphotropic Moloney murine leukemia virus (MoMLV) entry is mediated by the Ram-1 phosphate transporter.[4] Following fusion and entry, retroviruses reverse transcribe their RNA genomes to double stranded DNA in the cytoplasm of infected cells.[3] The DNA then moves to the nucleus for integration into the genomic DNA of the infected cell. Once integrated the 'provirus' utilizes the host cell machinery for transcription and translation of mRNAs to viral proteins. Integration is semirandom.[5] Encapsidation signals termed (E) target unspliced viral RNA genomes for incorporation into newly forming nucleocapsids at the inner cell membrane.[3] Completion of the viral life cycle occurs with budding of progeny virions from the host cell.[3]

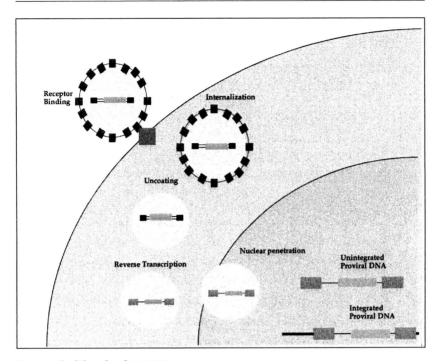

Fig. 4.1. The lifecycle of MoMLV.

Retroviral Gene Organization

All replication competent retroviruses encode for at least three essential viral gene products expressed as precursor polyproteins: Gag (group specific antigen) forms the viral capsid structural proteins, Pol (polymerase) encodes for reverse transcriptase, integrase and viral protease, and Env (envelope) encodes for the surface glycoprotein which mediates host cell viral attachment and fusion.[3] Retroviral RNAs are flanked by short repetitive sequences (R) and unique (U5 and U3) sequences at their 5' and 3' ends. During reverse transcription these sequences are duplicated to form the long terminal repeats (LTRs). The LTRs contain cis-acting sequences required for expression of viral genes and integration of proviral DNA. Other key cis-acting sequences lie between the LTRs and the *gag pol env* open reading frame and include the plus and minus strand primer binding sites essential for reverse transcription.[3]

Recombinant Retroviral Vectors

To date retroviral vectors based on the Moloney murine leukemia virus (MoMLV) have been used extensively in clinical trials because their biology is well understood and they offer the potential for long term expression from an integrated transgene.[2] By design they do not require the introduction of viral genes and therefore are unlikely to elicit immunity in the human host.[6,7]

Figure 4.2 illustrates the genomic organization of MoMLV. Gene transfer vectors based upon MoMLV are routinely engineered to retain the minimal amount of viral sequence required in cis for reverse transcription and integration of vector DNA, including the LTRs and a RNA encapsidation packaging signal (ψ+) extending into the gag open reading frame (Figure 4.2B).[6,7] Most vectors also contain a positive selectable marker gene in addition to a therapeutic gene of interest. Marker genes facilitate selection and enrichment of vector containing cells ex vivo and allow gene transfer and expression, e.g., transduction, to be monitored.[8] Recombinant retrovirus stocks are produced by transfection of the vector DNA into cell lines specifically engineered to express the deleted viral genes in trans, e.g. packaging cell lines (Fig. 4.3).[9,10] Traditional packaging cell lines for MoMLV-based vectors are derived from the mouse fibroblast cell line NIH3T3.[10-12] More recently, several groups have developed transient packaging systems based on the human embryonic kidney cell line 293.[13-17] This cell line can be transfected at high efficiency, resulting in vector titers comparable to those obtained following prolonged selection of stable packaging cell lines. Infectious retroviral vectors obtained from packaging cell lines are capable of infecting target cells but are unable to replicate further in the absence of viral genes. In short, preparations of MoMLV-based retrovirus vectors containing up to eight kilobases of heterologous DNA can readily be produced free of replication competent virus.

The major limitation to MoMLV-derived retroviral vector systems is their dependence on cell division for vector integration and stable transgene expression.[5] In addition, the relatively low titer of current MoMLV-based vectors results in inefficient gene transfer into hematopoietic target cells. Although MoMLV-based vectors have been used in a number of clinical gene transfer protocols aimed at genetic modification of human lymphocytes, prolonged culture ex vivo has been required to obtain useful numbers of transduced cells.[2,18] Moreover, transduction of hematopoietic progenitor cells with

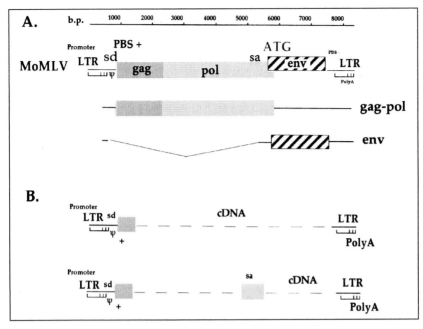

Fig. 4.2. Genomic structure of MoMLV and MoMLV based vectors. A. Schematic illustration of wild type Moloney murine leukemia virus (MoMLV) from which most recombinant retroviral vectors are derived. The virus contains three genes, gag, *pol*, and *env*, flanked by long terminal repeats (LTRs) which contain the viral promoter/enhancer sequences, integration sequences, and polyadenylation signals. B. Prototype vectors derived from murine viruses consist of replication defective recombinant genomes in which most of the retroviral genes have been replaced by the gene or genes to be introduced to the target cells. Most vectors retain the minimal cis-acting regions demonstrated to be required for viral replication and efficient transgene expression. LTRs provide essential cis-acting sequences for the synthesis and integration of proviral DNA, in addition to the viral promoter. Other cis-acting sequences include the plus and minus strand primer binding sites for the initiation of reverse transcription and extended ψ (encapsidation/dimerization) sequences (noted as ψ on figure) which allow vector transcripts to be incorporated into viral particles.

MoMLV-based vectors ex vivo requires the addition of growth factors which promote cell division.[18] As a result, transduction of primitive progenitor cells with MoMLV-based vectors may compromise the long term repopulating potential of this subset of cells.[18] To address these limitations, a number of strategies are being pursued for enhancing the efficiency and applicability of MoMLV-based gene transfer systems.

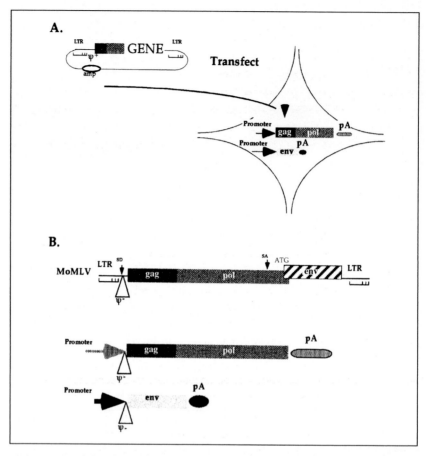

Fig. 4.3. Retroviral vector packaging lines. A. Packaging cell lines are engineered to express viral gene products in trans but lack the cis-acting ecapsidation (ψ) sequences necessary for inclusion of viral RNA into infectious particles. When recombinant vector genomes containing th etransgene are transfected in to these packaging cell lines, the cells produce recombinant virions containing the vector genome but no replication competent helper virus. The efficiency and safety of vector packaging is dependent on the extent to which these cis and trans-acting processes can be isolated. B. Illustration of first generation helper virus constructs and more recent technology for providing helper virus genes in trans. Early packaging cell lines were engineered with deleted ψ (encapsidation) signals, yet retained the wild type cis elements (e.g., LTRs) common to introduced vectors. Hence, a single recombination event between helper and vector genomes would lead to replication competent vectors. One approach for circumventing helper virus formation is to split the helper virus genome such that *gag pol* are expressed from one mRNA and *env* from another. Further, utilization of heterologous transcription initiation and termination signals reduces the amount of sequence shared between the transducing vector and helper genomes.

Vector Host Range

One strategy for increasing MoMLV-based vector titers and transduction efficiencies in human cells is by redirecting the host range of the virus by inclusion of heterologous envelope glycoproteins. Most MoMLV-based vectors used in human gene transfer protocols have utilized amphotropic murine leukemia virus (MLV-A) envelopes due to the broad distribution of its cognate receptor on human cells.[2] Replacing the wild type MoMLV envelope with an amphotropic envelope is one example of vector pseudotyping. The source of the envelope in such phenotypically mixed virions—in which the genome of one virus is encapsidated within the envelope of a different virus—is commonly referred to as the vector pseudotype. Another example is the utilization of the G protein of vesicular stomatitis virus (VSV-G) for pseudotyping MoMLV vectors.[19-22] VSV-G exhibits greater stability than amphotropic envelopes and VSV-G psuedotypes can be concentrated to high titer by centrifugation. For example, Sharma and coworkers recently reported enhanced transduction of tissue culture cells and peripheral blood leukocytes (PBL) using a VSV-G pseudotyped MoMLV-based retroviral vector.[22] At equivalent multiplicities of infection (MOI) the VSV-G pseudotyped vector showed a 22-fold increase in transduction efficiency on Jurkat cells relative to MLV-A. Furthermore, the efficiency of PBL infection mediated by the VSV-G pseudotyped vector increased linearly with increasing MOI to a maximum of 16-32% at an MOI of 40.[22] Similarly, other groups have reported on the ability of gibbon ape leukemia virus (GALV) envelopes for enhancing MoMLV based gene transfer into hematopoietic cells.[23-25] However, most of these studies resulted in only modest (2-fold) increase in gene transduction efficiencies over the widely used MLV-A. More interesting for HIV gene therapy is work by Mammano and colleagues. These authors recently developed an HIV-1-Env pseudotyped MoMLV-based vector.[26] Successful pseudotyping of the vector required truncation of the cytoplasmic domain of HIV-1-Env glycoprotein, gp41. Transduction of Hela-CD4 indicator cells was, on the average, several fold lower for the HIV-1-env pseudotype relative to MLV-A.[26] However, the potential for targeting the HIV-1-Env pseudotyped MLV-based vector to CD4-positive T cells by direct injection into the patient would greatly advance gene therapy strategies aimed at reducing HIV replication.

Expression of Anti viral Genes

Efficacious antiviral gene therapy requires that therapeutic genes be efficiently expressed in the relative hematopoietic target cells. Both RNA polymerase II-based (pol II) and RNA polymerase III-based (pol III) promoter systems are currently being utilized for expression of both RNA based and protein based antiviral genes. Expression of RNA based therapeutics requires efficient expression, folding, stabilization and trafficking to cellular compartments for colocalization with targets. Several groups have recently published experiments on the effect of vector design for expressing RNA based therapeutics (Fig. 4.4).[27,28] Most of these studies indicate that the presence of RNA pol III promoters in the U3 region of the 3' LTR (e.g., double copy vector) results in higher levels of chimeric RNA expression compared to when the RNA pol III promoter is internal to the viral LTRs, (e.g., single copy). For example, Gervaix and co-workers quantitated chimeric pol III derived transcripts obtained from vectors containing either one copy, two copies, or three copies of the RNA pol III promoter.[27] Estimation of chimeric RNA expression as quantitated by RT PCR was on average 1000-fold higher from triple copy vectors relative to double copy designs. Moreover, expression from double copy RNA pol III promoters was 1000-fold greater than single copy designs, and the level of HIV inhibition following HIV challenge was commensurate with RNA transcript levels when a chimeric RNA decoy/ribozyme was expressed from the pol III promoters.[27] In another study, Peng and coworkers constructed a series of retroviral vectors in which antisense RNAs were expressed from the viral LTR pol II promoter or from single and double copy RNA pol III promoters.[28] Following HIV challenge of vector transduced cell lines, the antisense inhibitor genes that were expressed from the double copy pol III promoter afforded more protection against HIV replication than did identical vectors in which the antisense RNA was expressed as part of the LTR pol II transcript.

Lentiviral Vectors

Another approach for targeting retroviral vectors to both circulating and tissue associated CD4+ T lymphocytes for which HIV is tropic is by utilization of an HIV-1 based vector. There are several advantages to such an approach. First, the presence of wild type HIV would result in rescue of the vector and subsequent spread and delivery of gene based antivirals to uninfected cells.[29] Second, in con-

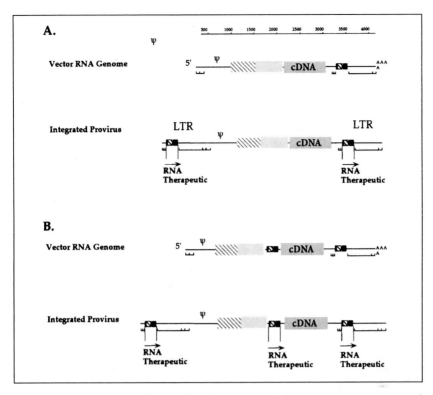

Fig. 4.4. Examples A and B illustrate 'double copy' proviral vector genomes engineered for delivery of RNA-based therapeutics. In example A the vector genome is engineered to contain a chimeric pol III-based expression cassette within the unique 3' end of the genome. Following reverse transcription, the U3 segment containing the pol III cassette becomes duplicated to the 5' LTR, resulting in a 'double copy' vector. In example B the vector genome carries additional copy of the pol III-based promoter internal to the viral LTRs.

trast to murine retroviral vectors in which stable transduction is dependent on cell division, vectors based upon HIV efficiently enter and integrate into noncycling cells.[29] This feature is of particular interest for transduction of terminally differentiating monocytes and macrophages for which HIV is tropic. More importantly, the ability to efficiently transduce nonproliferating primitive hematopoietic progenitor cells would greatly enhance HIV gene therapy strategies aimed at immune reconstitution through transduction of this subset of cells. Hence, development of lentiviral-based vectors has enormous potential for human gene transfer protocols aimed at immune reconstitution in AIDS.

HIV Vector Design

To date several vector systems based upon HIV-1 and HIV-2 have been described.[29-35] Critical to the development of safe and efficient lentiviral vectors is the identification of cis-acting RNA sequences responsible for encapsidation of the viral RNA genome into infectious particles. Deletion mapping studies have identified sequences believed important for encapsidation and dimerization of HIV-1 viral RNA.[30,31] HIV-1 encapsidation sequences are believed to begin 5' of the major splice donor site and extend into gag, much like MoMLV. However, it is unclear if other sequences within the HIV-1 genome contribute to efficient packaging of the viral RNA.[30,31]

Early attempts aimed at development of HIV-1-based gene delivery systems were hampered by the inability to establish stable packaging cell lines.[29] Therefore, a number of laboratories subsequently developed transiently-based expression systems for generating replication defective HIV vectors. For example, Naldini and colleagues developed a three-plasmid 293T transient transfection system consisting of a transducing vector and packaging components modeled on the split genome design common to MoMLV gene delivery systems.[32] The vector host range used in their studies was extended by pseudotyping with either amphotropic MLV or VSV-G envelope glycoproteins. The pseudotyped vectors were capable of transducing cell cycle arrested fibroblast and primary human macrophages, and in all cases exhibited enhanced transduction of nonproliferating cells relative to the MLV-A. Furthermore, transduction was shown to be dependent on a functional integrase gene, implying that transgene expression is dependent on integration of the vector into the host genome.[32] Other groups have also reported efficient transduction of noncycling primitive hematopoietic progenitor cells using VSV-G pseudotyped HIV-1 vectors.[30,35] In contrast to Naldini and co-workers, the HIV-1 vectors utilized for these studies were based upon a two plasmid transient transfection expression system. Two plasmid systems were constructed by engineering a marker gene in place of the wild type envelope sequence within a molecular clone of HIV.[30] Heterologous envelopes were then supplied in trans by cotransfection on a separate plasmid. Although suitable for proof of principle, the inclusion of viral gene products in cis to the vector genome limits the applicability of these vectors due to immunogenicity. More recently, Corbeau and coworkers described a stable HeLa packaging cell line based on a duotropic (e.g., T tropic and monocyte/macrophage tropic) molecular clone of HIV-1.[33] Vector supernatants obtained from this packaging cell line showed titers of 10[5] TU/ml on HeLa-T4 cell lines, and virus preparations were demonstrated to be free of replication competent retrovirus. The potential for in vivo targeting of these vectors to CD4+ lymphocytes and other hematopoietic cells tropic for HIV is encouraging.

Adeno-Associated Virus Gene Delivery Systems

Taxonomy
The adeno-associated viruses (AAV) of humans are naturally replication defective, nonpathogenic members of the Parvoviridae family of animal viruses.[34] These viruses have historically been classified into the autonomous and dependovirus subgroups according to their dependence on helper virus for replication.[34]

Life Cycle
In the absence of helper virus, human AAV establishes latent infection by site specific integration on the q arm of chromosome 19.[34] Super infection of latently infected cells by helper virus of either herpes virus or adenovirus families results in excision and replication of the AAV genome and the production of viral progeny.[34] Wild type AAV efficiently enters nondividing cells and exhibits a broad host range of infection.[34] To date, 5 serotypes of AAV have been described, but to date most vectors are based upon the well characterized AAV type 2.[37]

Genome Organization
Figure 4.5 illustrates the proviral genomic organization of AAV-2. The AAV genome consist of a 4.68 kilobase single-stranded DNA flanked by palindromic inverted terminal repeats (ITR).[37] The ITR serves as both the origin and primer for viral replication in addition to the encapsidation signal.[35] The virus contains two open reading frames (*rep* and *cap*) and three promoters named according to their approximate map positions in the proviral genome.[34] The *rep* genes are expressed from the p5 and p19 major promoters and encode for viral proteins involved in virus replication.[34] The *cap* genes are expressed from the major p40 promoter and encode for the viral structural proteins.[34] All mRNAs terminate at a single polyadenylation signal. Gene expression is dependent on helper virus mediated

transactivation of the AAV p5 and p19 promoters.[34] Subsequent synthesis of the Rep proteins permits transactivation of the p40 promoter and expression of the viral Cap structural genes.[34]

Adeno-Associated Virus-Based Vectors

Gene transfer vectors based on AAV are promising for gene therapy due to their potential for site specific integration into a broad range of noncycling mammalian cells. The minimal wild type AAV sequence requirement for generation of replication defective AAV-based vectors is the inverted terminal repeats (ITR).[34,36,37] Deletion of the viral genome and promoters permits insertion of up to 5 kilobase of heterologous DNA.[36] Most vectors require heterologous transcriptional control elements for expression of a transgene of interest. Although it is clear that the *rep* gene product is required for site specific integration, most vectors used to date do not contain a functional *rep* gene, due to cytotoxitiy associated with its expression.

Typically, replication defective AAV is produced by co-transfecting a transducing vector containing the gene of interest with packaging plasmids providing the AAV *rep* and *cap* genes in trans.[34,37] Cells are then super infected with helper virus (e.g., adenovirus) resulting in the generation of both AAV and adenovirus progeny.[34,37] AAV virions containing the transgene, but no helper virus genomes, can be purified by cesium chloride density centrifugation or by heat inactivation of adenovirus.[34,37] Similar to retroviral gene delivery systems, packaging plasmids are designed to minimize vector and helper sequence homology to minimize chance recombination.

Although there remains much uncertainty regarding the stability of AAV-based gene delivery, recent evidence suggest that these vectors may be effective at stably transducing noncycling target cells ex vivo. Podsakoff and coworkers recently described an AAV-derived vector capable of efficiently entering nonproliferating tissue culture cells ex vivo.[38] Tissue culture cells (line 293 and human diploid fibroblasts) were arrested by treatment with chemical DNA synthesis inhibitors or by serum starvation followed by transduction with an AAV-based vector. Gene transfer as monitored by LacZ expression was equivalent to or greater in arrested cells as compared to actively dividing controls. Following a 100,000-fold expansion of the cell cultures without selection, vector specific DNA was demonstrated by Southern blot analysis to be integrated into high molecular weight chromosomal DNA.[41] The authors speculate that the vector DNA in

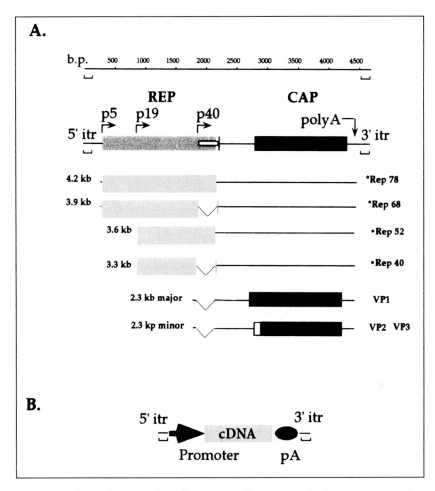

Fig. 4.5. A. Schematic illustration of AAV proviral genome and mRNAs. AAV has a linear single stranded 4.6 κb DNA genome flanked by palindromic inverted terminal repeats, (ITRs). The viral genome is transcribed from three major promoters, p5, p19, and p40, producing 7 primary transcripts. AAV genomes are divided into two distinct coding regions, *rep* (replication) and *cap* (capsid). The *rep* gene encodes for at least 4 polypeptides involved in replication and *cap* encodes for at least 3 capsid polypeptides. B. Examples of AAV-derived recombinant vector genomes. The minimal wild type sequences required in cis for generation of recombinant AAV-based vectors are the inverted terminal repeats (ITRs). Most vectors are designed to contain heterologous promoters and polyadenylation sequences for expression of a transgene of interest.

an episomal form may have integrated after release of the proliferative block. However, the result of these experiments suggests that AAV vectors can efficiently infect nondividing cells and persist until integration. Another report by Inouye et al used an AAV-based vector for transfer of HIV specific inhibitors into primary CD4

T lymphocytes and terminally differentiated alveolar macrophages for which HIV is tropic.[39] Transduction of greater than 40% of activated CD4-positve T cells was achieved and reported stable for the length of the experiment (e.g., 4-6 weeks). In addition, transduction of nondividing alveolar macrophages as monitored by LacZ expression exceeded 90%. Following HIV challenge, both cell types transduced with AAV vectors expressing gene based antivirals exhibited potent resistance to HIV replication.[39]

Conclusions

In summary, intracellular immunization is in principle an important gene therapy based approach for treating AIDS. Recent understanding of the magnitude of HIV-1 turnover and capacity for rapid mutation necessitates the development of gene transfer technology that will result in the prolonged and sustained expression of genetic therapies. Currently, three viral delivery systems, murine retroviral vectors, lentiviral vectors and AAV vectors, all have promising properties as well as drawbacks. Ultimately, chimeric vectors with characteristics of each of these systems may be developed.

References

1. Baltimore D. Gene therapy intracellular immunization. Nature 335; 1988:395.
2. Crystal R. Transfer of genes to humans: early lessons and obstacles to success. Science 270; 1995:404-410.
3. Levy JA ed.*The Retroviridae.* Plenum Press, New York, NY, 1992.
4. Miller D. Cell-surface receptors for retroviruses and implications for gene transfer. Proc Natl Acad Sci 93; 1996:11407-11413.
5. Miller D, Adam M, Miller A. Gene transfer by retrovirus vectors occurs only in cells that are actively replicating at the time of infection. Mol Cell Biol 1990;10:4239-4242.
6. Armentano D, Yu S, Kantoff P, von Ruden T, Anderson F, Gilboa E. Effect of internal viral sequences on the utility of retroviral vectors. J Virol 1987; 61:1647-1650.
7. Miller A, Rosman G. Improved retroviral vectors for gene transfer and expression. Biotechniques 1989; 7:980-990.
8. Phillips K, Gentry T, McCowage G, Gilboa E, Smith C. Cell-surface markers for assissing gene transfer into human hematopoietic cells. Nature Medicine 1996; 2:1154-1156.
9. Mann R, Mulligan R, Baltimore C. Construction of a retroviral packaging mutant and its use to produce helper free defective retrovirus. Cell 1983; 33:153-159.

10. Miller A, Buttimore C. Redesign of retrovirus packaging cell lines to avoid recombination leading to helper virus production. Mol Cell Biol 1986; 6:2895-2902.

11. Markowitz D, Goff S, Bank A. Construction and use of a safe and efficient amphotropic packaging cell line. Virology 1988; 167:400-406.

12. Markowitz D, Goff S, Bank. A safe packaging line for gene tranfer: Separating viral genes on two different plasmids. Journal of Virology 1988; 62:1120-1124.

13. Finer M, Dull T, Qin L, Farson D, Roberts M. kat: a high efficiency retroviral transduction system for primary human T lymphocytes. Blood 1994; 83:43-50.

14. Landau N, Littman D. Packaging system for rapid production of murine leukemia virus vectors with variable tropism. J Virol 1992; 66:5110-5113.

15. Pear W, Nolan G, Scott M, Baltimore D. Production of high-titer helper free retroviruses by transient transfection. Proc Natl Acad Sci USA 1993; 90:8392-8396.

16. Naviaux R, Costanzi E, Haas M, Verman I. The pCL Vector system: Rapid production of helper-free, high-titer, recombinant retroviruses. Journal of Virology 1996; 70:5701-5705.

17. Soneoka Y, Cannon P, Ramsdale E, Griffiths J, Romano G, Kingsman S, Kingsman A. A transient three-plasmid expression system for the production of high titer retroviral vectors. Nucleic Acids Research 1995; 23:628-633.

18. Hanania E, Kavanagh J, Hortobagyi G, Giles R, Champlin R, Deisseroth A. Recent advances in the application of gene therapy to human disease. The American Journal of Medicine 1995; 99:537-552.

19. Emi N, Friedmann T, Yee J-K. Pseudotype formation of murine leukemia virus with the g protein of vesicular stomatitis virus. Virol 1991; 65:1202-1207.

20. Ory D, Neugeboren B, Mulligan R. A stable human-derived packaging cell line for production of high titer retrovirus/vesicular stomatitis virus G pseudotypes. Proc Natl Acad Sci USA 1996; 93:11400-11406.

21. Schnell M, Buonocore L, Kretzschmar E, Johnson E, Rose J. Foreign glycoproteins expressed from recombinant vesicular stomatitis viruses are incorporated efficiently into virus particles. Proc Natl Acad Sci USA93; 1996:11359-11365.

22. Sharma S, Cantwell M, Kipps T, Friedmann T. Efficient infection of a human T cell line and of human primary peripheral blood leukocytes with a pseudotyped retrovirus vector. Proc Natl Acad Sci USA 1996; 93:11842-11847.

23. Bauer T, Miller D, Hickstein D. Improved transfer of the leukocyte integrin cd18 subunit into hematopoietic cell lines by using retroviral vectors having a gibbon ape leukemia virus envelope. Blood 1995; 86:2379-2387.

24. Porter C, Collins M, Tailor C, Parkar M, Cosset F, Weiss R, Takeuchi Y. Comparison of efficiency of infection of human gene therapy target cells via four different retroviral receptors. Human Gene Therapy 1996; 7:913-919.
25. von Kalle C et al. Increased gene transfer into human hematopoietic progenitor cells by extended in vitro exposure to a psuedotyped retroviral vector. Blood 1994; 84:2890-2897.
26. Mammano F, Salvatori F, Indraccolo S, Rossi A, Chieco-Bianchi L, Gottlinger H. Truncation of the human immunodeficiency virus type 1 envelope glycoprotein allows efficient pseudotyping of moloney murine leukemia virus particles and gene transfer into cd4+ cells. Journal of Virology 1997; 71:3341-3345.
27. Gervaix A, Li X, Kraus G, Wong-Staal F. Multigene antiviral vectors inhibit diverse human immunodeficiency virus type 1 clades. Journal of Virolgoy 1997; 71:3048-3053.
28. Peng H, Callison D, Li P, Burrell C. Long-term protection against HIV-1 infection conferred by tat or rev antisense RNA was affected by the design of the retroviral vector. Virology 1996; 220:377-89.
29. Parolin C, Sodroski J. A defective HIV-1 Vector for gene transfer to human lymphocytes. Journal of Molecular Medicine 1995; 73:279-288.
30. Akkina R, Walton R, Chen M, Li Q, Planelles V, Chen I. High-efficiency gene transfer into CD34+ cells with a human immunodeficiency virus type 1-based retroviral vector pseudotyped with vesicular stomatitis virus envelope glycoprotein G. Journal of Virology 1996; 70:2581-2585.
31. Carroll R et al. A human immunodeficiency virus type 1 (HIV-1)-based retroviral vector system utilizing stable HIV-1 packaging cell lines. J Virol 1994; 68:6047-51.
32. Corbeau P, Kraus G, Wong-Staal F. Efficient gene transfer by a human immunodeficiency virus type 1 (HIV-1)-derived vector utilizing a stable HIV packaging cell line. Proc Natl Acad Sci USA 1996; 93:14070-5.
33. Naldini L et al. In vivo gene delivery and stable transduction of nondividing cells by a lentiviral vector. Science 1996; 272:263-267.
34. Page K, Landau N, Littman D. Construction and use of a human immunodeficiency virus vector for analysis of virus infectivity. Journal of Virology 1990; 64:5270-5276.
35. Reiser J, Harmison G, Kluepfel-Stahl S, Brady R, Karlsson S, Schubert M. Transduction of nondividing cells using pseudotyped defective high-titer HIV type 1 particles. Proc Natl Acad Sci USA 1996; 93:15266-15271.
36. Lever A, Gottlinger H, Haseltine W, Sodroski J. Identification of a sequence required for efficient packaging of human immunodeficiency virus type 1 RNA into virions. Journal of Virology 1989; 63:4085-4087.
37. Muzyczka N. Use of adeno-associated virus as a general transduction vector for mammalian cells. Curr Top Microbiol Immunol 1992; 158:97-129.

38. Linden R, Ward P, Giraud C, Winocour E, Berns K. Site-specific integration by adeno-associated virus. Proc Natl Acad Sci USA 1996; 93:11288-11294.
39. Flotte T, Carter B. Adeno-associated virus vectors for gene therapy. Gene Ther 1995; 2:357-62.
40. Flotte T, Barraza-Ortiz X, Solow R, Afione S, Carter B, Guggino W. An improved system for packaging recombinant adeno-associated virus vectors capable of in vivo transduction. Gene Ther 1995; 2:29-37.
41. Podsakoff G, Wong K, Chatterjee S. Efficient gene transfer into non-dividing cells by adeno-associated virus-based vectors. Virol 1994; 68:5656-5666.
42. Inouye R et al. Potent inhibition of human immunodeficiency virus type 1 in primary T cells and alveolar macrophages by a combination anti-rev strategy delivered in an adeno-associated virus vector. Virol 1997; 71:4071-4078.

CHAPTER 5

T Lymphocyte Based HIV Gene Therapy Strategies

Tracy Gentry

Introduction

Diseases of the immune system have been the primary focus of gene therapy strategies targeted to T lymphocytes. These diseases include adenosine deaminase deficiency (ADA), purine nucleoside phosphorylase deficiency (PNP), leukocyte adhesion deficiency (LAD), and chronic granulomatus disease (CGD).[1] Other disease states have also become candidates for gene therapy approaches such as treatment of tumors through modification of tumor infiltrating lymphocytes.[2,3] The treatment of viral diseases including HIV, EBV and CMV infection with gene modified T lymphocytes is another area of intense research.[4-19,57] T cells are attractive target cells for gene therapy strategies because they are easy to obtain from the peripheral blood and are relatively easy to expand, select and characterize.[1,21-23]

Vectors for Gene Transfer into T Lymphocytes

Retroviral Vectors

As described in chapter 4, many delivery systems have been developed to introduce genes into T lymphocytes; each comes with its own set of advantages and disadvantages. Retroviruses continue to be the vector of choice for gene delivery to cells of the hematopoietic system, including T lymphocytes.[1] Retroviral vectors allow for stable integration of the genetic material into the host genome. This is critical in treatment of most T lymphocyte disorders where long-term expression of the inserted gene product is required.[1,22,23] In addition, retroviral vectors have a high efficiency of gene transfer and expression in many hematopoietic cell types.[1,22] The primary disadvantages of retroviral vectors include the inability to fully characterize the vector preparations due to their production in cultured cells, the risk of activating oncogenes via insertional mutagenesis or transcriptional activation of oncogenes downstream from the integrated retrovirus, production of replication competent retrovirus in the vector preparations, and a requirement that cells be actively dividing for efficient integration of the vector.[1,22] As described in chapter 2, a number of groups have demonstrated that retroviral vectors encoding HIV inhibitors can stably transduce T cell lines and inhibit replication and expression of HIV.[5,12,13,16,17]

Adeno-Associated Viral Vectors

Adeno-associated virus (AAV) is a nonpathogenic DNA virus that may not require cell proliferation for infection.[24, 25,26] Wild-type AAV integrates into a specific region of chromosome 19, but integration in this region seems to occur less frequently with recombinant AAV vectors.[24] The primary limitations in using AAV for T cell gene transfer strategies are the packaging limit of the AAV virion and the difficulty of vector production and purification. Several groups have used AAV to introduce HIV inhibitory genes into immortalized CD4+ T lymphocytes. Chatterjee et al demonstrated stable gene transfer into T cell lines with AAV vectors encoding anti-sense RNA to HIV as well as potent inhibition of HIV replication.[26] Smith et al showed that no deleterious effects were seen in cell growth or CD4 expression in CEM-SS cells transduced with AAV vectors expressing RRE and TAR decoys (see chapter 2), and no significant rearrangements of the vector were observed in long term transduced cells.[27] When CEM-SS cells were challenged with HIV, viral replication and expression was inhibited as effectively in cells transduced with AAV vectors expressing the RRE and TAR decoys as in cells transduced with retroviral vectors expressing the same RRE and TAR decoys. Intriguingly, there seemed to be some inhibition of HIV by a control AAV vector not expressing any RNA inhibitors, indicating that AAV itself may have some HIV inhibitory activity.

Adenoviral Vectors

Adenovirus has a wide host range of infection and low pathogenicity in humans.[28] As with AAV, adenovirus can introduce genetic material into nonreplicating cells. Abe et al demonstrated that CD8+ T lymphocytes transduced with an adenoviral vector expressing γ-interferon reduced the tumor burden more effectively than control CD8+ T lymphocytes in a preclinical animal model.[30] Another study using adenovirus to introduce IL-2 into tumor-specific T lymphocytes achieved 100% cell transduction efficiencies as compared to 1% transduction efficiencies achieved with retroviral vectors. Mice treated with the IL-2 gene modified tumor infiltrating lymphocytes (TILs) survived longer than controls or mice treated with nongene modified TILs.[31] Adenovirus, however, has distinct disadvantages for HIV gene therapy purposes. Adenoviral vectors do not appear to stably integrate into the host genome and consequently, vector expression decreases as the transduced cells proliferate.[28,29] Another disadvantage of adenoviral vectors is that many of the viral genes are included.[22] This leads to potent immune responses to adenoviral proteins expressed in the infected cells and relatively rapid immune mediated destruction of adenoviral transduced cells.

Liposome/DNA Complexes

In addition to viral based gene delivery systems, liposomes complexed with DNA (lipofection) have also been used to deliver genes to T cells. Liposomes are noninfectious and appear nonimmunogenic in vivo.[32] Lipofection has been used more frequently in cancer immunotherapy, where only short term gene expression is required, than in gene therapy for acquired or infectious diseases where stable long-term expression is desired. However, Philip et al reported the development of a technique involving lipofection of plasmid DNA containing elements of AAV that resulted in long-term expression in transfected T lymphocytes (>30 days).[32] Maximum gene expression was seen between days 2-7; by day 15 gene expression had declined but remained stable up to 25 days. This approach could ultimately be useful for obtaining high level, long term expression in T lymphocytes while avoiding the complications of viral vector systems.

Adenoviral Assisted Transfection

A variation on lipofection is adenoviral-assisted transfection.[33-35] This method involves noncovalently complexing DNA to an extracellular ligand such as transferrin or a polycation such as polylysine. The DNA complex is then further complexed to adenovirus. The extracellular ligand functions to bind the DNA/adenoviral complex to membrane receptors, where it is endocytosed. Following endocytosis, the adenovirus functions to inactivate lysosomes so that the DNA complex escapes degradation. Kelleher et al demonstrated that this technique could result in stable gene transfer in human lymphoblastoid cell lines.[34] Merwin et al directed DNA delivery to T cells using an antibody to CD5 complexed with polylysine, DNA, and adenovirus.[33] In another example, transferrin was replaced with an antibody to CD3 by Buschle and colleagues to deliver genes specifically to T cells.[35] Binding of the DNA/adenoviral complex was specific to T cells, but expression was transient. The gene transfer efficiency with this vector was 50% in cell lines, and 5% in primary T cells. Adenoviral-assisted transfection has also been used to introduce HIV inhibition genes including a TAR decoy, an antisense gag transcript, and a dominant negative mutant of gag into a T cell line.[10] Gene transfer efficiencies of 60-90% were reported and gene expression was maintained for 2 weeks.

Particle Bombardment

Another nonviral approach to introducing genes into T lymphocytes is via particle bombardment. Particle bombardment relies on physical force to deliver DNA, and thus is less dependent on uptake mechanisms than many of the gene delivery approaches described above.[36] Several particle bombardment systems have been developed. One of these involves using high-velocity micro projectiles to deliver DNA into intact cells and tissues from a hand-held biolistic system that employs gunpowder containing bullets for discharge. Mouse tissues bombarded with tungsten coated DNA particles using this system demonstrated gene transfer efficiencies of 25% with stable gene expression maintained for 2 weeks.[37] Another method of particle bombardment uses high voltage electric discharge to generate a shock wave which accelerates DNA-coated gold particles to high velocity so that they penetrate the cell membrane. A 3% gene transfer efficiency was observed in T cells following gene transfer with this method.[36] Woffendin and colleagues compared particle bombardment gene transfer to retroviral transduction in T lymphocytes using vectors encoding HIV inhibitors including RevM10.[4] Retrovirally transduced T cells had a gene transfer efficiency of 0.1-10% that increased to 10-60% after G418 selection. In comparison, particle bombardment gene transfer efficiencies were approximately 3%, increasing to greater than 50% after selection. Upon challenge with HIV, the inhibition of viral spread was similar in cells genetically modified with particle bombardment and retroviral vector transduction. An advantage to particle bombardment over retroviral transduction in HIV gene therapy is that T cell activation can be avoided. This could minimize activation of HIV in autologous T cells and could preserve the biologic properties of the manipulated T lymphocytes.

Improving Retroviral Vector Gene Transfer Efficiency in T Lymphocytes

While many of the gene transfer strategies described above may ultimately be useful for T cell based HIV gene therapies, retroviral vectors remain the vehicle of choice for achieving long-term stable gene expression. Consequently, many groups have explored methods to improve gene transfer into T lymphocytes using these vectors. Achieving high efficiency retroviral gene transfer into T lymphocytes will most likely be dependent both on vector biology and T cell biology. For example, vector titer and the type of vector envelope could play critical roles in determining the T cell gene transfer efficiency. In addition, the proliferative status of the T cell may also be a critical determinant of the gene transfer efficiency. Lastly, simple physical issues such as the ratio of virus to cell, the temperature of transduction, and other variables could also play important roles in the efficiency of gene transfer.

In order to investigate the role that each of these issues plays in T cell gene transfer, it is critical to accurately and sensitively measure the gene transfer efficiency. Until recently, the majority of retroviral vectors that have been described in the literature used the neomycin phosphotransferase gene as a marker for gene transfer. Gene transfer efficiency with this gene is estimated using G418 selection and/or DNA analysis. There are several disadvantages to using these methods to measure gene transfer efficiency. G418 selection takes 7-14 days, it is difficult to quantitate the proportion of transduced cells which survive selection, and G418 selection compromises the growth of T cells. DNA-based techniques such as 'semiquantitative' PCR or DNA blotting are cumbersome, inaccurate, and potentially misleading. For example, DNA analysis could overestimate the gene transfer efficiency if transduced cells harbor more than one copy of DNA. In addition, DNA analysis may detect vector fragments, unintegrated virus, and nonfunctional proviruses.

To address these issues, Mavilio et al, as well as a number of other groups, have developed a variety of marker genes which express cell surface proteins, such as the nerve growth factor receptor (NGFR), which can be detected in transduced cells by immunofluorescence staining.[39-45] The frequency of transduced cells can then be rapidly enumerated using FACS analysis (Fig. 5.1). Transduced cells can also be isolated easily by FACS or physical methods.[42,44] The development of vectors expressing cell surface markers, and other in situ markers including β-galactosidase and green fluorescence protein(GFP), has made it relatively easy to screen and identify conditions that improve gene transfer into CD4 enriched T cells.[21,45,46]

Cocultivation of T Lymphocytes with Retroviral Vector Producer Cells

Cocultivation has traditionally been the most effective method for achieving high efficiency retroviral vector transduction of T lymphocytes and other cells. This method involves incubating the T cells to be transduced directly on the retroviral packaging cell lines. Strair et al reported 50-100% gene transfer efficiencies using a LacZ expressing vector in primary T lymphocytes, and reported that mitogenic stimulation of the cells did not appear to improve the gene transfer efficiency.[38] Other groups have also reported high levels of gene transfer into T cells using coculture.[21,30,58] However, despite the high levels of gene transfer, this method is not desirable for clinical applications due to the risk of infusing a patient with packaging cells and technical difficulties in isolating T lymphocytes from the packaging cell monolayers.[21,40]

Optimizing Gene Transfer into T lymphocytes with Retroviral Vector Supernatants

Due to the drawbacks of coculture transduction techniques, many groups have focused on ways to improve retroviral vector transduction using vector supernatants obtained from the packaging lines. We conducted a study to systematically evaluate the effect that opti-

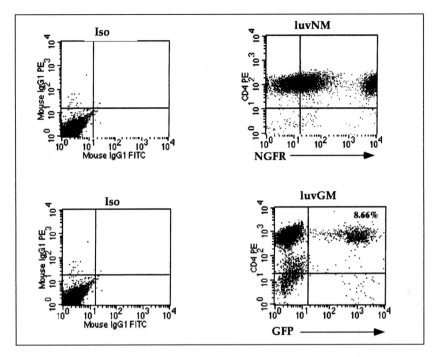

Fig. 5.1. Gene transfer into CD4+ T lymphocytes using the NGFR and GFP marker genes with retroviral vectors luvNM expresses NGFR, luvGM expresses GFP.

mizing physical parameters would have on the gene transfer efficiency in peripheral blood CD4+ T lymphocytes.[21] First, we analyzed what effect alternative T cell mitogens and the length of mitogen stimulation would have on gene transfer efficiency. Using an NGFR expressing vector, we found that gene transfer efficiency was 3- to 5-fold higher when cells were mitogen stimulated for 48 hours prior to transduction compared to shorter or longer times. Next, we compared transduction using PHA to transduction using soluble anti-CD3 and/or soluble anti-CD28. The gene transfer efficiency using a combination of soluble anti-CD3 and soluble anti-CD28 was similar to slightly better than PHA and significantly better than using anti-CD3 alone as was done in most previous studies.

Other physical factors that we examined in this study included the length of time of exposure of T cells to viral supernatant, the number of target cells per milliliter of viral supernatant, the viral supernatant dilution, the effects of centrifugation of the T cells with viral supernatant, and the effects of multiple transductions. A slight increase in the gene transfer efficiency was observed as the length of time during which the cells were incubated with viral supernatant was increased from 30 minutes to 12 hours. No substantial differences were observed with further incubation beyond 12 hours. A modest increase in gene transfer efficiency was seen as the T cell concentration was progressively lowered from 10^7 cells/ml of viral supernatant to 10^5 cells/ml. The gene transfer efficiency was similar in T cells regardless of whether viral supernatant was undiluted or progressively diluted up to 1 part in 4. Since dilution of viral supernatant reduces some of the logistical difficulties and safety concerns inherent in generating large volumes of retroviral supernatants, this is a useful observation. Kotani et al reported that centrifugation of cells with retroviral supernatant at 2500 rpm for 90 minutes increased gene transfer efficiency 4- to 18-fold in a variety of cell types.[47] Bunnell and colleagues also have reported improved gene transfer efficiency using centrifugation.[48] Similarly, we observed a 3- to 5-fold increase in gene transfer efficiency in peripheral blood CD4+ T lymphocytes when using centrifugation. Multiple exposures of cells to retroviral supernatants also doubled the gene transfer efficiency as reported by others.[5,7,16,17] Combining all of the improved conditions identified above resulted in a retroviral supernatant-based gene transfer procedure that routinely yields a gene transfer efficiency of 25-40% in peripheral blood lymphocytes as opposed to the 1-3% gene transfer efficiencies obtained prior to optimizing these physical parameters.[21]

Fibronectin

A recently described procedure for improving retroviral transduction that appears promising is the use of fibronectin in the gene transfer cultures. Three binding sites on fibronectin that participate in cell adhesion have been identified. These are the heparin binding domain which interacts via cell surface molecules; the CS1 sequence which mediates adhesion via the VLA-4 integrin; and the cell binding domain which mediates adhesion via the VLA-5 integrin. Since retroviral particles bind to sequences within the heparin binding domain and hematopoietic cells may bind to the other domains, the addition of fibronectin to the gene transfer cultures may increase the physical proximity of the vector virions to the target cells. The transduction efficiency of human hematopoietic progenitor cells has been substantially increased by using chymotryptic fragments of fibronectin.[40] Gene transfer efficiency was 50-75% in human hematopoietic progenitor cells after a one day exposure to retrovirus while adherent to a fibronectin fragment that contained all three cell

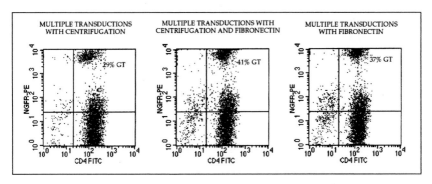

Fig. 5.2. Effect of centrifugation and fibronectin treatment on the retroviral vector gene transfer efficiency in peripheral blood CD4+ T lymphocytes. GT=gene transfer efficiency.

adhesion sites. In contrast, the gene transfer efficiency was reduced to baseline levels if either the binding sites for the retrovirus or the cells were deleted from the fibronectin molecule. This method of transduction may alleviate the need for polycations, cocultivation, and extended in vitro exposure to growth factors. In preliminary studies within our lab, the addition of the fibronectin fragment to the gene transfer cultures replaces the need for centrifugation but does not add to the gene transfer efficiencies currently obtained (Fig. 5.2)

Additional Potential Methods for Improving Retroviral Vector Gene Transfer into T Lymphocytes

Combining Retroviral Vectors and Liposomes

Combining liposomes composed of cationic and neutral lipids with retroviral vectors has been shown to enhance retroviral transduction >60-fold compared to retrovirus alone into a human fibrosarcoma cell line.[49] In comparison, polybrene, a polycation frequently employed to increase the gene transfer efficiency, gave a 10-fold increase over virus alone. Mixing polybrene and liposomes with the retroviral vectors did not increase gene transfer efficiency further. It is thought that the increased gene transfer efficiency using this approach is due to charge neutralization by the lipids, suggesting that liposomes act through the same mechanism as polybrene, only more efficiently. Currently, neither we nor others have reported that this procedure improves the retroviral vector gene transfer efficiency in primary T lymphocytes; however, studies comparing alternative liposomes and transfection conditions are underway.

Combining Retroviral Vectors and Calcium Phosphate Precipitation

Morling and colleagues demonstrated that coprecipitating retroviral vectors with calcium phosphate could improve transduction efficiency.[50] In initial experiments, they demonstrated that a two hour incubation of cells with viral supernatant resulted in removal of only 5% of the virus from the media, indicating that the majority of retroviral vector virions in the supernatant were not taken up by the target cells. When calcium chloride ($CaCl_2$) was added, a precipitate containing calcium phosphate and viral particles developed in less than 30 minutes. After precipitation, less than 1% of the virus remained in the supernatant. Transduction efficiency could then be increased by either precipitating the viral supernatant and adding this to the cells or by adding the calcium chloride to the cells and then adding the retroviral supernatant. Improved transduction efficiencies were seen on all the human cell lines tested, including an epidermoid carcinoma, bladder carcinoma, colon carcinoma, and a B cell lymphoma. Improved transduction efficiencies for primary T cells using this method have not yet been reported, but, again, studies are underway to test this strategy.

Flow Through Transduction

Since it appears that the majority of the virus in the viral supernatants never come into contact with target cells during transduction, Chuck and colleagues developed a "flow through transduction" procedure.[51] Since vector virions move by Brownian motion, based on the limited movement and the half-life of the virus, only those viral particles in physical proximity to the cells will ever be capable of transduction. The limitations of Brownian motion can be overcome by directing the motion of the virus to the cells. One way to accomplish this directed motion is by fluid flow of the retroviral supernatant through a porous membrane that supports the target cells. Using NIH 3T3 cells as the target cells on collagen coated culture inserts, higher gene transfer efficiencies were observed with the flow-through method than with static transduction. Flow-through transduction also overcomes some of the technical issues that complicate retroviral transduction for clinical applications. It has led to higher transduction efficiencies even at low virus concentration, thus eliminating concerns associated with production of high-titer viral supernatant. Flow-through transduction also does not require the use of polycations such as polybrene or protamine to enhance the gene transfer efficiency. Studies to optimize retroviral gene transfer into T cells using flow through transduction are underway in our laboratory and others.

Clinical Trials Involving Gene Transfer into T Lymphocytes

To date, several gene therapy trials have been reported which involve genetic modification of T lymphocytes. In general, the goals of these studies were to determine the safety and feasibility of this approach to treating diseases.

Severe Combined Immune Deficiency due to Adenosine Deaminase Deficiency(ADA-SCID)

Patients enrolled in some of the first clinical gene therapy trials for ADA-SCID involving infusions of gene modified T lymphocytes are now up to 35 months post-treatment. In a trial conducted in Italy, 2 patients were treated with gene therapy after failing ADA enzyme replacement therapy.[52] Two retroviral vectors encoding ADA, differing in their restriction enzyme digestion pattern, were used in this study so that the source of the gene modified cells could be determined. One ADA encoding vector was transduced into autologous peripheral blood lymphocytes (PBLs) and the other vector was used to transduce autologous bone marrow cells (BM). One patient received 7.2 x 10^8 transduced lymphocytes and 3.5 x 10^7 transduced BM cells in 9 intravenous infusions over 24 months. The second patient received slightly less cells in 5 infusions over 10 months. Analysis for the persistence of the transduced cells was done at monthly or bimonthly intervals. Six months after treatment, survival of the vector transduced cells was seen in both patients. During the early time points after the infusions, transduced cells were predominantly derived from a pool of long-lived PBLs. However, after one year following treatment, the relative concentration of transduced PBLs derived from the gene modified bone marrow began increasing, indicating that bone marrow derived gene modified T cells were capable of longer term survival than gene modified PBLs. Gene corrected ADA producing cells also demonstrated a survival advantage over ADA deficient cells and administration of transduced cells restored some facets of immune function in both patients. No toxicity from the therapy was indicated, and the presence of helper virus was not detected. This study, while on limited numbers of patients, did demonstrate that gene therapy treatment for ADA-SCID was feasible and safe. Whether clinical efficacy was achieved remains unclear.

In a second clinical trial involving treatment of ADA-SCID with gene modified peripheral blood T cells conducted at the National Institutes of Health in the United States, feasibility and safety was also demonstrated.[20] Autologous PBLs were transduced with an ADA encoding retroviral vector and infused multiple times. Again, the transduced cells appeared to have a selective survival advantage over nontransduced cells. One patient has had a normal T cell count for two years since the last infusion of gene modified T cells and the proportion of circulating T cells that contained the vector remained stable. A second patient demonstrated some improvement in several aspects of immune function as well.

Epstein Barr Virus (EBV) Associated Lymphoproliferative Disorders (LPDs)

Heslop and colleagues have been exploring the effectiveness of administering EBV specific cytotoxic T cells (CTLs) to patients undergoing bone marrow transplant who develop EBV-LPDs or who are at high risk for this disorder.[19,53-55] In these studies, EBV-specific CTLs were prepared, transduced with a retroviral vector encoding the neomycin phosphotransferase gene, and infused into ten allograft recipients at high risk for EBV LPDs. No clinical toxicity was noted. In three patients with evidence of EBV reactivation, EBV DNA concentrations (which had increased 1000-fold) returned to control range within 3-4 weeks. One patient who developed an immunoblastic lymphoma achieved a complete remission (CR) following administration of EBV-specific CTLs. Gene marked T cells were identified in several recipients for prolonged periods of time and, interestingly, the numbers of gene marked T cells increased in some cases coincident with reactivation of EBV. This indicated that the gene marked EBV-CTLs may have been responding to EBV activation by proliferation and expansion. These studies have provided important insights into the biology of adoptively transferred cytotoxic T cells and provide the foundation for future studies designed to optimize the persistence and activity of these cells.

HIV Infection

Woffendin and colleagues used particle bombardment of HIV inhibitors into autologous T cells to address the feasibility of gene therapy for treatment of HIV infection.[57] In their clinical trial, 3 patients were treated. Peripheral blood mononuclear cells were leukapheresed, CD8 depleted, transduced by particle bombardment with RevM10 or a negative control with an efficiency of approximately 10%, and expanded in vitro for 10 days prior to infusion. Patients received equal numbers of cells transduced with either RevM10 or the negative control. The patients were initially infused with 10^9 cells, but patients 2 and 3 had subsequent infusions of 2×10^{10} cells after no recombinant genes were found even 1 hour after infusion of 10^9 cells. When 2×10^{10} cells were infused, equal numbers of RevM10 transduced cells and negative control cells were seen 1 hour after infusion. One week after infusion the relative ratio of RevM10 to control was increased 10-fold. Patient 3 maintained detectable RevM10 cells up to 8 weeks, and these cells demonstrated a 4- to 5-fold selective survival advantage. It was also observed that no new abnormalities resulted from treatment and the levels of serum p24 and HIV RNA did not increase. These results demonstrate the feasibility and safety of T cell mediated gene therapy in HIV infection and indicate that HIV genetic inhibitors may provide a survival advantage to gene modified T lymphocytes.

Greenberg, Riddell and colleagues have been conducting an elegant series of studies designed to optimize the activity of adoptively transferred CMV and HIV specific cytotoxic T lymphocytes (CTLs) in immunocompromised patients.[56] In order to be able to eliminate the infused CTLs if they cause deleterious effects, HIV CTLs were transduced with a retroviral vector encoding the herpes virus thymidine kinase (TK) gene which confers sensitivity to the drug Gancyclovir. Consequently, gene modified T cells could be eliminated by administration of Gancyclovir to the patient. The vector also encoded (as a fusion to the TK gene) the hygromycin phosphotransferase (Hy) gene in order to positively select transduced T cells in vitro prior to infusion into the patients. Five of the first six patients infused with these gene modified CTLs developed potent cellular immune responses against the hybrid HyTK protein expressed in the transduced cells.[56] These results indicate that retroviral vector gene products can be potent immunogens and that consideration of this issue is critical to successful retroviral gene transfer into T lymphocytes and other cells.

Summary

In summary, gene therapy using modified T lymphocytes is evolving into a means of treatment for some diseases, including HIV infection. However, there are still many challenges to be addressed, including further improving the gene transfer efficiency in T lymphocytes, optimizing the function of the gene modified cells and eliminating vector mediated immunogenicity. Many improvements, particularly in the retroviral vector system, have been made that have increased gene transfer efficiency from a few percent to 20-40% in primary T cells. But in systems where the cells do not have a selective survival advantage, even this level of gene transfer may not be adequate to achieve clinically relevant levels of gene modified T cells within patients. Development of new and/or improved vector systems, as well as techniques to manipulate and expand primary T cells ex vivo, inevitably will lead to improvements in the clinical utility of this gene therapy strategy.

References

1. Cournoyer D. Gene therapy of the immune system. Annu Rev Immunology 1993; 11:297-329.
2. Nash M, Platsoucas C, Wong B, Wong P, Cottler-Fox M, Otto E, Freedman R. Transduction of rIL-2 expanded CD4+ and CD8+ ovarian TIL-derived T- cell lines with the G1Na (neo^R) replication-deficient retroviral vector. Human Gene Therapy 1995; 6:1379-1389.
3. Hwu P, Rosenberg S. The genetic modification of T cells for cancer therapy: an overview of laboratory and clinical trials. Cancer Detection and Prevention 1994; 18(1):43-50.
4. Woffendin C, Yang Z, Udaykumar R, Xu L, Yang N, Sheehy M, Nabel G. Nonviral and viral delivery of a human immunodeficiency virus protective gene into primary human T cells. Proc Natl Acad Sci USA 1994; 91:11581-11585.
5. Leavitt M, Yu M, Yamada O, Gunter K, Looney D, Poeschla E, Wong-Staal F. Transfer of an anti-HIV-1 ribozyme gene into primary human lymphocytes. Human Gene Therapy 1994; 5:1115-1120.
6. Sun LQ, Pyati J, Smythe J, Wang L, Macpherson J, Gerlach W, Symonds G. Resistance to human immunodeficiency virus type 1 infection conferred by transduction of human peripheral blood lymphocytes with ribozyme, antisense, or polymeric trans-activation response element constructs. Proc Natl Acad Sci USA 1995; 92:7272-7276.

7. Vandendriessche T, Chuah M, Chiang L, Chang L, Ensoli B, Morgan R. Inhibition of clinical human immunodeficiency virus (HIV) type 1 isolates in primary CD4+ T lymphocytes by retroviral vectors expressing anti-HIV genes. Virol 1995; 69(7):4045-4052.

8. Duan L, Zhu M, Bagasra O, Pomerantz R. Intracellular immunization against HIV-1 infection of human T lymphocytes: utility of anti-Rev single-chain variable fragments. Human Gene Therapy 1995; 6:1561-1573.

9. Yamada O, Yu M, Yee J, Kraus G, Looney D, Wong-Staal F. Intracellular immunization of human T cells with a hairpin ribozyme against human immunodeficiency virus type 1. Gene Therapy 1994; 1:38-45.

10. Lori F, Lisziewicz J, Smythe J, Cara A, Bunnag T, Curiel D, Gallo R. Rapid protection against human immunodeficiency virus type 1 (HIV-1) replication mediated by high efficiency nonretroviral delivery of genes interfering with HIV-1 tat and gag. Gene Therapy 1994; 1:27-31.

11. Pomerantz R, Trono D. Genetic therapies for HIV infections: promise for the future. AIDS 1995; 9:985-993.

12. Sullenger B, Gallardo H, Ungers G, Gilboa E. Overexpression of TAR sequences renders cells resistant to human immunodeficiency virus replication. Cell 1990; 63:601-608.

13. Lee S, Gallardo H, Gilboa E, Smith C. Inhibition of human immunodeficiency virus type 1 in human T cells by a potent Rev response element decoy consisting of the 13-nucleotide minimal Rev-binding domain. Virol 1994; 68(12):8254-8264.

14. Shaheen F, Duan L, Zhu M, Bagasra O, Pomerantz R. Targeting human immunodeficiency virus type 1 reverse transcriptase by intracellular expression of single chain variable fragments to inhibit early stages of the viral life cycle. Virol 1996; 70(6):3392-3400.

15. Miele G, Lever A. Expression of mutant and wild-type gag proteins for gene therapy in HIV-1 infection. Gene Therapy 1996; 3:357-361.

16. Plavec I et al. High transdominant RevM10 protein levels are required to inhibit HIV-1 replication in cell lines and primary T cells: implication for gene therapy of AIDS. Gene Therapy 1997; 4:128-139.

17. Lisziewicz J, Sun D, Lisziewicz A, Gallo R. Antitat gene therapy: a candidate for late-stage AIDS patients. Gene Therapy 1995; 2:218-222.

18. Caputo A et al. Inhibition of HIV-1 replication and reactivation from latency by tat transdominant negative mutants in the cysteine rich region. Gene Therapy 1996; 3:235-245.

19. Culver K et al. Lymphocytes as cellular vehicles for gene therapy in mouse and man. Proc Natl Acad Sci USA 1991; 88:3155-3159.

20. Blaese R et al. T lymphocyte-directed gene therapy for ADA-SCID: Initial trial results after 4 years. Science 1995; 270:475-480.

21. Rudoll T et al. High-efficiency retroviral vector mediated gene transfer into human peripheral blood CD4+ t lymphocytes. Gene Therapy 1996; 3:695-705.

22. Miller D. Human gene therapy comes of age. Nature 1992; 357: 455-460.

23. Blaese R. Progress toward gene therapy. Clinical Immunology and Immunopathology 1991; 61:S47-S55.

24. Flotte T, Carter B. Adeno-associated virus vectors for gene therapy. Gene Therapy 1995; 2:357-362.

25. Muro-Cacho C, Samulski R, Kaplan D. Gene transfer in human lymphocytes using a vector based on adeno-associated viruses. Journal of Immunotherapy 1992; 11:231-237.

26. Chatterjee S, Johnson P, Wong K. Dual-target inhibition of HIV-1 in vitro by means of an adeno-associated virus antisense vector. Science 1992; 258:1485-1488.

27. Smith C et al. Transient protection of human T cells from human immunodefiency virus type 1 infection by transduction with adeno-associated viral vectors which express RNA decoys. Antiviral Research 1996; 32:99-115.

28. Kass-Eisler A, Falck-Pedersen E, Elfenbein D, Alvira M, Buttrick P, Leinwand L. The impact of developmental stage, route of administration and the immune system on adenovirus-mediated gene tranfer. Gene Therapy 1994; 1:395-402.

29. DeMatteo R et al. Gene transfer to the thymus: a means of abrogating the immune response to recombinant adenovirus. Annals of Surgery 1995; 222(3):229-242.

30. Abe J et al. In vivo antitumor effect of cytotoxic T lymphocytes engineered to produce interferon-ψ by adenovirus-mediated genetic transduction. Biochemical and Biophysical Research Communications 1996; 218(0029):164-170.

31. Nakamura Y et al. Adoptive immunotherapy with murine tumor-specific T lymphocytes engineered to secrete interleukin 2. Cancer Research 1994; 54:5757-5760.

32. Philip R et al. Efficient and sustained gene expression in primary T lymphocytes, and primary and cultured tumor cells mediated by adeno-associated viral plasmid complexed to cationic liposomes. Molecular and Cellular Biology 1994; 14(4):2411-2418.

33. Merwin J et al. CD5-mediated specific delivery of DNA to T lymphocytes: Compartmentalization augmented by adenovirus. Immunol Meth 1995; 186:257-266.

34. Kelleher Z, Vos J. Long-term episomal gene delivery in human lymphoid cells using human and avian adenoviral-assisted transfection. BioTechniques 1994; 17(6):1110-1117.

35. Buschle M et al. Receptor-mediated gene transfer into human T lymphocytes via binding of DNA/CD3 antibody particles to the CD3 T cell receptor complex. Human Gene Therapy 1995; 6:753-761.

36. Burkholder J, Decker J, Yang N. Rapid transgene expression in lymphocyte and macrophage primary cultures after particle bombardment-mediated gene transfer. Immunol Meth 1993; 165:149-156.

37. Hui K, Sabapathy T, Oei A, Chia T. Generation of allo-reactive cytotoxic T lymphocytes by particle bombardment-mediated gene transfer. Journal of Immunological Methods 1994; 171:147-155.
38. Strair R, Towle M, Heald P, Smith B. Retroviral mediated transfer and expression of exogenous genes in primary lymphoid cells: Assaying for a viral transactivator activity in normal and malignant cells. Blood 1990; 76(6):1201-1208.
39. Mavilio F et al. Peripheral blood lymphocytes as target cells of retroviral vector-mediated gene transfer. Blood 1994; 83(7):1988-1997.
40. Hanenberg H, Xiao X, Dilloo D, Hashino K, Kato I, Williams D. Colocalization of retrovirus and target cells on specific fibronectin fragments increases genetic transduction of mammalian cells. Nature Medicine 1996; 2(8):876-882.
41. Conneally E, Bardy P, Eaves CJ, Thomas T, Chappel S, Shpall EJ, Humphries RK. Rapid and efficient selection of human hematopoietic cells expressing murine heat-stable antigen as an indicator of retroviral-mediated gene transfer. Blood 1996; 87:456-64.
42. Medin JA et al. A bicistronic therapeutic retroviral vector enables sorting of transduced CD34+ cells and corrects the enzyme deficiency in cells from Gaucher patients. Blood 1996; 87:1754-62.
43. Planelles V, Haislip A, Withers-Ward ES, Stewart SA, Xie Y, Shah NP, Chen ISY. A new reporter system for detection of retroviral infection. Gene Therapy 1995; 2:369-376.
44. McCowage GB, Phillips KL, Gentry TL, Hull S, Kurtzberg J, Gilboa E, Smith C. Multiparameter FACS analysis of retroviral vector gene transfer into primitive umbilical cord blood cells. Experimental Hematology 1998; 26:288-298.
45. Phillips K, Gentry T, McCowage G, Gilboa E, Smith C. Cell-surface markers for assessing gene transfer into human hematopoietic cells. Nature Medicine 1996; 2(10):1154-1156.
46. Pawliuk R, Kay R, Lansdorp P, Humphries RK. Selection of retrovirally transduced hematopoietic cells using CD24 as a marker of gene transfer. Blood 1994; 84:2868-77.
47. Kotani H et al. Improved methods of retroviral vector transduction and production for gene therapy. Human Gene Therapy 1994; 5:19-28.
48. Bunnell BA, Muul LM, Donahue RE, Blaese RM, Morgan RA. High-efficiency retroviral-mediated gene transfer into human and non-human primate peripheral blood lymphocytes. Proc Natl Acad Sci 1995; 92:7739-7743.
49. Hodgson C, Solaiman F. Virosomes: Cationic liposomes enhance retroviral transduction. Nature Biotechnology 1996; 14:339-342.
50. Morling F, Russel S. Enhanced transduction efficiency of retroviral vectors coprecipitated with calcium phosphate. Gene Therapy 1995; 2:504-508.
51. Chuck A, Palsson B. Consistent and high rates of gene transfer can be obtained using flow-through transduction over a wide range of retrovial titers. Human Gene Therapy 1996; 7:743-750.

52. Bordignon C et al. Gene therapy in peripheral blood lymphocytes and bone marrow for ADA-immunodeficient patients. Science 1995; 270:470-475.
53. Heslop HE et al. Administration of neomycin-resistance-gene-marked EBV-specific cytotoxic T lymphocytes to recipients of mismatched-related or phenotypically similar unrelated donor marrow grafts. Human Gene Therapy 1994; 5:381-97.
54. Heslop HE et al. Long-term restoration of immunity against Epstein-Barr virus infection by adoptive transfer of gene-modified virus-specific T lymphocytes. Nature Medicine 1996; 2:551-5.
55. Rooney CM et al. Use of gene-modified virus-specific T lymphocytes to control Epstein-Barr-virus-related lymphoproliferation. Lancet 1995; 345:9-13.
56. Riddell SR et al. T cell mediated rejection of gene-modified HIV-specific cytotoxic T lymphocytes in HIV-infected patients [see comments]. Nature Medicine 1996; 2:216-23.
57. Woffendin C, Ranga U, Yang Z, Xu L, Nabel G. Expression of a protective gene prolongs survival of T cells in human immunodeficiency virus-infected patients. Proc Natl Acad Sci USA 1996; 93:2889-2894.
58. Finer M, Dull T, Qin L, Farson D, Roberts M. *kat*: A high efficiency retroviral transduction sytstem for primary human T lymphocytes. Blood 1994; 83(1):43-50.

CHAPTER 6

Stem Cell-Based Gene Therapies in the Treatment of AIDS

Robert Storms

Introduction

A cquired immune deficiency syndrome (AIDS) is a slow, progressive disease that debilitates immune function. AIDS has a viral etiology where cells, predominantly hematopoietic cells that express the CD4 surface antigen, become infected with the type 1 human immunodeficiency virus (HIV). HIV is a small, enveloped RNA virus that belongs to the lentivirinae subfamily of retroviruses. The lentiviruses, in general, give rise to progressive disease states in their infected hosts. As a retrovirus, HIV replicates through the reverse transcription of its RNA genome into a double stranded DNA element which then integrates into the genome of infected cells. Thus, cells that survive the initial infection become persistently infected with HIV. From a therapeutic standpoint it may therefore be helpful to consider that individuals infected with HIV are essentially genetic mosaics, where some of their somatic cells carry a pathogenic genetic element. At this level, AIDS may be viewed as a genetic disease and may therefore be treatable through the emerging technologies of gene therapy.

This review intends to detail strategies for gene therapies that might be implemented against the HIV virus. In particular, a focus will be placed on those strategies that might be administered within the context of bone marrow transplantation using gene-modified hematopoietic stem cells. These therapies are highly speculative, particularly in the face of the recent successes in pharmacological treatments for AIDS. The gene therapies for AIDS are pursued largely

Gene Therapy for HIV Infection, edited by Clay Smith. © 1998 Springer-Verlag and R.G. Landes Company.

with the realization that, with the extreme adaptability of this virus, HIV variants will probably evolve to resist the current drug therapies. The problems faced by HIV gene therapy strategies are those faced by stem cell-based gene therapies in general. Thus, the limitations to the success of these therapies to date will be evaluated within the larger context of our current knowledge of hematopoietic stem cell biology.

The HIV Life Cycle and Antiviral Therapies

The pathophysiology of AIDS has been widely reviewed (see chapter 1).[1] The treatment of AIDS is complicated by the fact that many cells infected with HIV do not die. Unlike diseases arising from lytic viruses (e.g., polio), some HIV-infected cells survive the initial infection to actively produce virus for prolonged periods. Still other HIV-infected cells establish latent reservoirs where the virus lies dormant until reactivated at some later time. It is these latent reservoirs of virally infected cells that make AIDS such a problematic syndrome for treatment. Indeed, the therapies currently available for the treatment of AIDS attempt to ablate active production of virus but cannot address the more fundamental problems presented by persistent, latent viral infection.

Two unique aspects of HIV replication have been targeted in the pharmacological antiviral therapies currently available.[2,3] The strategy most widely used disrupts viral DNA synthesis. As mentioned previously, the HIV genome is packaged in the virion as RNA. Prior to integration into the host cell genome, this RNA is reverse transcribed into double stranded DNA by an RNA-dependent DNA polymerase (reverse transcriptase). Several agents (e.g., AZT, ddI, ddC and D4T) disrupt viral DNA synthesis. These agents are dideoxynucleotide analogs that incorporate into DNA but fail to be extended. DNA synthesis therefore halts upon their incorporation. The dideoxynucleotide analogs are used preferentially by the viral reverse transcriptase; however, they are likewise bound by cellular DNA polymerases with low efficiency. As a result, each of these drugs exhibits mild, tissue specific cytotoxic effects for the patient. Fortunately, each of these agents exhibits unique cytotoxicities and the patient may be rotated through drug regimens to reduce damage to specific tissues. The rotation through multiple drug regimens also reduces the likelihood of selecting HIV variants that are resistant to one specific drug. A second target for anti-HIV therapies has been the viral protease. Like other retroviruses, the HIV virus synthesizes its structural proteins as polyproteins which are then cleaved into smaller proteins prior to their assembly into the virus particle.[2] The viral protease used for this processing is sufficiently unique to make it an excellent target for antiviral therapy. In clinical trials, inhibitors of this protease have proven strikingly effective in reducing patients' viral burdens, particularly when administered in conjunction with the dideoxynucleotide analogs and other drugs.[4,5]

Since integrated viruses are never killed by these drugs, AIDS patients must be diligent in maintaining their treatments. Each time the virus is permitted to expand, the probability of escape mutation increases and drug resistant variants of HIV could be selected. When these drugs are used individually the probability of selecting such escape mutations is relatively high, and perhaps even inevitable. Escape mutations for the nucleotide analogs would require only a minor change in the affinity that the viral reverse transcriptase has for dideoxynucleotide analogs. Similarly, the generation of an HIV variant that is resistant to a protease inhibitor might require only a subtle change in the affinity of the protease for its inhibitor. The risk of escape mutations has been reduced by using these drugs in combination. In this scenario, the mutations required to entirely escape the therapy would require two independent events, each of which would follow a single hit dynamic.

HIV as a Target for Gene Therapy

Gene therapy is currently being explored as a form of antiviral therapy for HIV. In these therapies, inhibitors of HIV replication or integration would be placed into the genome of susceptible cells. Thus, gene therapies would provide "intracellular immunization," where cells acquire a stable, permanent resistance to infection by HIV.[6] One potentially suitable class of therapeutic genes would include those encoding dominant negative suppressor proteins. Dominant negative inhibition is possible when a protein functions within a multimeric complex of one or multiple species of proteins. The presence of a single dominant negative protein within a larger complex of proteins is sufficient to disrupt the normal function of the entire complex.

Two dominant negative inhibitor proteins have been characterized that could potentially provide resistance to HIV in a clinical setting. A dominant negative Gag protein can disrupt replication of

HIV in cultured cells.[7] The group-specific antigens (Gag) are the proteins that form the inner core of the virus particle.[2] Assembly of the core is entirely dependent upon the multimerization of the Gag proteins, and in the absence of this multimerization mature virus particles cannot be produced. A second dominant negative suppressor of HIV replication is a suppressor of Rev function.[8] The Rev protein binds a specific RNA sequence (located within the *env* gene) to facilitate the transport of those RNAs from the nucleus to the cytosol of the cell (reviewed in ref. 2). In this way the Rev protein enhances the translation of RNAs encoding viral structural genes.

One potential advantage of these agents is that it is likely that escape mutations from the dominant negative proteins are difficult to achieve. Since these proteins function through disrupting normal interactions, a reversion of phenotype would require that the wild type virus evolve to the point where the dominant negative protein is no longer disruptive. Viral escape mutants would require that the wild type protein either does not interact with the dominant negative protein or that the association of the dominant negative protein no longer disrupts the function of the entire protein complex.

The Gag and Rev dominant negative suppressor proteins may present the more difficult problem of delivering a target protein that elicits cytotoxic T lymphocytes (CTLs).[9] AIDS patients possess HIV-specific CTLs and therefore probably possess active CTLs against the Gag and Rev proteins.[1] Since dominant negative suppressor proteins are nearly identical to their normal counterparts, the cellular immune system will probably treat any cells expressing these proteins as foreign. Thus, as part of the process of eliminating HIV-infected cells, the immune response of HIV-infected patients may attack the therapeutic cells secondarily.

Nonprotein alternatives to the dominant negative suppressor proteins are available. Two essential HIV gene products bind RNA in a site-specific manner. Stated more precisely, two HIV proteins recognize specific stem-loop tertiary structures within the HIV genome. The Tat protein enhances transcription of all viral genes and facilitates the elongation of the RNAs encoding structural genes, while the Rev protein facilitates the transport of specific RNA species out of the nucleus (reviewed in ref. 2). Since both of these proteins recognize specific RNA structures, it has been possible to design small "decoy" RNAs to inhibit their function.[10,11] The Tat and Rev proteins exhibit a high affinity for the decoys. Thus, the expression of excess decoy RNA would competitively inhibit the function of the Tat or Rev protein.

The RNA decoys have distinct advantages in gene therapy applications. First, no translation is required. This means that one level of complexity for providing the stable expression of a foreign gene has been eliminated. Secondly, using currently available selection technologies it is possible to identify RNA sequences that bind the target protein with higher affinity than does the wild type sequence. Finally, the chances for escape mutations by HIV seem remote in that the HIV virus would require two independent and simultaneous mutations. The Rev or Tat protein would need to mutate to recognize a different RNA stem-loop structure and, simultaneously, the recognition site within the HIV RNA would need to mutate to the new sequence recognized by the Rev or Tat protein.

It is currently unknown whether the RNA decoys would serve as immunogens for cytotoxic T lymphocytes. Since the decoys themselves are highly structured, they might serve as immunogenic epitopes. Indeed, these RNA stem-loop structures have evolved for specific, high affinity interactions with proteins. Thus, it may be possible to elicit CTLs against RNA decoys. However, it is unlikely that CTLs specific for the RNA decoys would already be present in AIDS patients at the time that the therapy is initiated. This distinction from the dominant negative suppressor proteins is significant.

Candidate Cell Types for HIV Gene Therapy

To be of clinical relevance, the antiviral genes must be deliverable to a cell type that is a target for infection by HIV. The predominant clinical manifestation of AIDS is the lack of CD4+ T lymphocytes in the peripheral blood and lymph nodes. Thus, there are two appropriate cell types that may be useful for applying AIDS gene therapies: lymphocytes and hematopoietic stem cells. Each of these cell types has distinct advantages and disadvantages. Lymphocyte-based gene therapies are covered in more detail elsewhere in this volume. However, a brief exploration of the therapeutic value of lymphocytes may likewise illustrate the specific advantages of stem cell-based therapies.

Lymphocytes do offer distinct advantages in gene therapies.[12] First and foremost among these is that lymphocytes may be harvested and expanded rapidly ex vivo under very well defined conditions. These factors would certainly facilitate gene transfer into the appropriate target cells. Furthermore, their ex vivo expansion would permit the selection of transduced cells prior to their reinfusion into the patient. Thus, the patient could receive a highly enriched population of therapeutic cells. Lymphocytes are relatively long-lived and, once delivered, the infused cells would have a selective survival advantage. Lymphocyte-based therapies would require multiple re-infusions over the life of the patient; however, the ease with which the cells can be manipulated ex vivo may compensate for this.

The disadvantages of lymphocyte-based therapies are that, for multiple different reasons, these therapies would only partially restore immune function in the infected patient. While the primary target for HIV is CD4+ T cells, HIV infects other hematopoietic cells, particularly monocytes. In fact, in the establishment of a new infection there is an initial selection for HIV variants that exhibit a tropism for monocytes; it is only as the disease progresses that T-lymphotropic HIV variants are selected.[1] A greater concern would be that as lymphocytes are expanded ex vivo the repertoire of immune responsive cells is diminished, particularly if only gene-modified cells are selected and used for reinfusions. Finally, as mentioned previously, there is the clear possibility that gene-modified lymphocytes will be selectively killed by the patient's cellular immune response when reintroduced into the patient.

Most of the shortcomings of lymphocyte-based therapies can be addressed by using stem cell-based gene therapies. The one clear advantage of these strategies is that complete immune function could theoretically be reconstituted in the patient. A hematopoietic stem cell will, by definition, give rise to all hematopoietic lineages. Thus, the therapeutic gene would be present in both monocytic and lymphoid cells. In addition, as the stem cell differentiates into the lymphoid lineages it would provide a complete T cell repertoire. The immune reconstitution would require the prior cytoablation of the patient, thereby eliminating cytotoxic T lymphocytes that might exist in the periphery. Furthermore, in the process of re-education, the T cells arising from the transplant would not recognize the therapeutic cells as foreign.

Hematopoietic Stem Cells as Targets for Gene Therapy

A Hierarchy of Hematopoietic Cells

To apply stem cell-based gene therapies it is necessary to understand the fundamental biology of the hematopoietic stem cell. The hematopoietic system exists as a hierarchy of cells at varying stages of commitment and differentiation. This hierarchy permits rapid, plastic responses while preserving a reservoir of the most primitive cells. The hematopoietic cells can be partitioned into at least 3 broad classes of cells based on their potential to differentiate and on their capacity for self-renewal.[13,14] The most primitive cells are multilineage or pluripotent hematopoietic stem cells (HSC). These cells exhibit a high capacity for self-renewal and are the reservoir of the hematopoietic system for the entire life span of any animal. The HSC have the potential to differentiate into any of the major hematopoietic cell types (Fig. 6.1). Each cell division by an HSC involves a decision to either self-renew or to divide while committing to lineage-specific differentiation. When pluripotent stem cells differentiate they initially become committed or lineage-restricted hematopoietic progenitors. These cells are more abundant than HSC, have a more limited capacity for self-renewal than HSC, and are dedicated to differentiation into specific functional cells at the periphery. The final class of hematopoietic cells are terminally differentiated, functional cells with either highly limited or no capacity for self-renewal. These are far and away the most numerous hematopoietic cells.

To describe this hierarchy as clearly delineated cell types is convenient but misleading. For this discussion it is important to stress that intermediate stages of pluripotent progenitors have been described and the existence of these cells raises important considerations in the implementation of stem cell-based gene therapies.[15-19] These intermediate pluripotent cells are most evident as cells that contribute to multiple hematopoietic cell lineages immediately posttransplant, but which can not provide stable reconstitution of the hematopoietic system.[15-19] Thus, these cells are distinguishable in vivo by virtue of their diminished capacity for self-renewal. These exhaustible multipotent cells have been characterized through the transplantation of gene-modified, congenic or otherwise "marked" sources of bone marrow-derived stem cells in experimental settings. The progeny of "marked" stem cells can be analyzed to infer the in vivo behavior of individual clonal progenitors. Typically, cells of this intermediate class of multipotent cells are detectable through broad fluctuations in the clonal origin of cells that reconstitute the periphery. The durations of these clonal fluctuations appear to vary with the size and/or longevity of the animal used as a experimental model. In the murine model clonal fluctations persist for the first 4 to 6 months immediately posttransplant, while in feline models similar fluctations

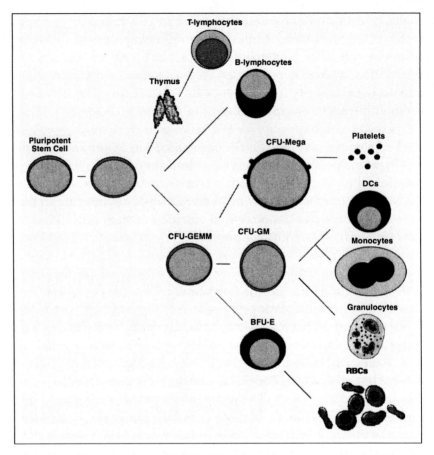

Fig. 6.1. The current hierarchical model of hematopoiesis.

are evident for 1 to 4.5 years.[15,17-21] Beyond these time frames the majority of pluripotent cells that persist appear to provide permanent engraftment and are therefore HSC.

Defining the Hematopoietic Stem Cell

Stem cell-based gene therapies rely on the modification of those pluripotent stem cells that will provide life-long contributions to hematopoiesis. This cell is the true HSC and its extreme scarcity imposes severe limitations on gene therapies. The evidence for a single cell capable of total hematopoietic reconstitution has been provided in multiple animal studies using limiting numbers of test cells in competitive repopulation assays.[14] It is significant that, in at least one human transplant recipient, clonal repopulation of the hematopoietic system was observed.[22] In humans, the frequency of the repopulating stem cell is unknown; however, an estimate of its frequency can be inferred from patients that obtained polyclonal reconstitution following allogeneic bone marrow transplants. One study estimated that, in 16 transplants, 116 ($\pm$ 40) reconstituting HSC were delivered when roughly 3×10^8 bone marrow-derived mononuclear cells/kg were transplanted.[23] If an average human mass is 70 kg, then the frequency of transplantable stem cells would be conservatively placed at 0.5 to 1 cell out of every 10^8 bone marrow-derived mononuclear cells. This frequency is much lower than that estimated for either murine or feline bone marrow. This estimate is likewise consistent with the concept that the frequency of HSC decreases with the size and/or longevity of the animal.

Hematopoietic stem cell biology is further complicated by the lack of a defined phenotype for isolating HSC. There are currently no selectable phenotypes to distinguish exhaustible pluripotent progenitor cells from the stem cells that would provide long-term, stable reconstitution. Human multipotent hematopoietic cells have been described with the CD34+ phenotype; however, this simple phenotype is broad and also encompasses diverse species of lineage-restricted progenitors.[24-36] More primitive subpopulations of CD34+ cells can be isolated by eliminating cells that express surface antigens typically associated with specific cell lineages or antigens that are generally associated with cell differentiation (e.g., CD38, CD33, or CD71).[15,25,26,28-31] To date, most of the work on human hematopoietic stem cells has focused on these subpopulations of CD34+ cells. It is important to note here that, although these cell populations may be rigorously purified, they still represent a diverse mixture of cell types.

The Evaluation of Human Hematopoietic Stem Cell Function

One other obstacle in studies on the HSC is a lack of reliable in vitro assay systems available to evaluate its function. The two most commonly used in vitro culture assays both quantify myelo-erythroid progenitors. Clonogenic myelo-erythroid progenitors can be enumerated by their growth in methylcellulose supplemented with cytokines in the hematopoietic progenitor colony assay (HPCA).[37] Cells of these lineages form well defined colonies that may be scored either as hematopoietic progenitor colonies or as colony forming cells with high proliferative potential (HPP-CFC). The HPP-CFC and

HPCA are committed myeloid progenitors and not HSC. More primitive subsets of hematopoietic progenitors are detectable by first supporting their growth on bone marrow-derived stromal monolayers for 5 weeks prior to performing an HPCA.[38-40] Cells that initiate long-term stromal cultures (*long-term culture-initiating cells* or LTC-IC) are a rare subset of hematopoietic cells that will not form assayable colonies directly upon their isolation, but only after their differentiation in vitro. Thus, one parameter for the isolation of HSC might include obtaining cell populations enriched for LTC-IC that likewise lack the more mature clonogenic progenitors.

Most cell culture systems are two dimensional and static and therefore do not mimic the bone marrow, where functional HSC are maintained for a lifetime. In vitro culture systems have now been developed to imitate the structure of the bone marrow.[41,42] In these cultures the cells expand within a three dimensional lattice and are fed by the continuous perfusion of media through this space. When perfusion chambers are seeded with cells from whole bone marrow the cultures establish a balanced mixture of cells of diverse lineages, and the proportions of these cell populations are maintained for extended periods of time. These cultures are currently being used to explore the possibility of expanding HSC ex vivo; where the perfusion cultures would be initiated from a single bone marrow and the stem cells from that marrow expand within a milieu of its own cells. Eventually these cultures may prove invaluable for monitoring gene transfer into HSC.

It is possible that in vitro cultures, no matter how sophisticated, may not support the true HSC. Instead, these cultures may merely select for cells capable of growth under artificial in vitro conditions. This has provided impetus to develop in vivo experimental models for human HSC function. The animal models most commonly used are mice with severe combined immune deficiency (SCID).[43] For expanding human hematopoietic cells these animals typically require small segments of human fetal bone, thymus or liver tissue to be embedded under the mouse kidney capsules. Human hematopoietic cells home to these tissues and differentiate. One mouse model, the NOD SCID mouse, permits the engraftment of human cells directly into the bone marrow of the mouse provided the mice are injected with a regimen of human cytokines. This model has led to the definition of a new hematopoietic progenitor designation, the SCID repopulating cell or SRC.[30,44,45] These cells may be the earliest progenitor assayable in an experimental system. The SCID animal models provide elegant means for elucidating the ontogeny of human hematopoietic lineages, although it is still uncertain whether these models are a truly accurate reflection of an authentic transplant setting.

Gene Therapy Using Hematopoietic Stem Cells

The ultimate goal for stem cell-based gene therapies is to deliver corrective genes to HSC, and then to provide this cell to patients in a transplant setting. The challenge of these strategies is to deliver genes to HSC without destroying their potential for long-term engraftment in the bone marrow. Foreign genes have been successfully delivered to HSC in murine bone marrow transplant models.[17-19,46-48] These murine studies provide valuable proofs of principle for the stem cell-based gene therapies. Most importantly, they validate that foreign genes can be delivered to an HSC without destroying its potential to reconstitute a transplant recipient. These cells behave in all respects as normal HSC: They reconstitute all hematopoietic lineages and have a very high potential for self-renewal. Indeed, gene-modified HSC have been serially transplanted into secondary recipient mice, where they still maintain the potential for multilineage development.[18]

The preliminary work targeting gene transfer into human hematopoietic progenitors has been encouraging. Clonogenic hematopoietic progenitors and LTC-IC have been transduced with relatively high efficiency using a variety of gene transfer conditions.[49-53] However, to date only a few studies have been performed that would permit an evaluation of gene transfer into reconstituting HSC in humans or nonhuman primates. Unfortunately, the results of these studies have been less encouraging. Very limited engraftment of gene-modified stem cell preparations have been documented in these trials.[54-57] Typically, fewer than 1% of peripheral blood cells are derived from gene-modified progenitors. Taken together, these findings would suggest that the conditions for gene delivery have been optimized for short-lived hematopoietic progenitors that do not provide long-term reconstitution.

In the absence of a larger number of studies, the limitations to the success of the stem cell-based gene therapies can only be evaluated in terms of the potential pitfalls within the protocols themselves. The protocols for gene transfer that are currently in clinical use may all be simplified as three stage processes that involve:

1. an enrichment of a HSC pool from a larger body of cells;
2. the ex vivo culture and transduction of the HSC pool in the presence of cytokines; and,
3. the transplantation of the gene-modified pool of cells. As will be discussed, many of the likely weaknesses of stem cell-based gene therapies may lie within the process of cell selection and the subsequent gene transduction.

The Enrichment of Hematopoietic Stem Cells for Gene Transfer

The transduction of murine HSC can be accomplished without any initial enrichment steps. The enrichment for pools of cells containing human HSC is pragmatic and largely driven by the need to transduce cells with clinical grade stocks of retroviral supernatants. These virus stocks are typically low titer and therefore large volumes would be required without some form of prior HSC enrichment. An absolute purification of HSC is currently unachievable and it should be noted that any enrichment for HSC likewise enriches for hematopoietic progenitors at many different stages of development. These progenitor subsets complicate the interpretation of data intended to estimate gene delivery into HSC.

Most strategies for the enrichment of HSC involve a positive selection for cells that express CD34. The use of CD34 as a selective marker has been based on the demonstration that a subset of these cells exhibits the potential for multilineage development both in vitro and in chimeric animal models. The CD34+ cells are a diverse population that include multipotent cells as well as lineage restricted progenitors. Indeed, when human CD34+ cells are transplanted without gene modification, they provide stable, continuing multilineage hematopoietic development for at least up to 1 year.[58,59] Similarly, the engraftment of gene-modified CD34+ HSC preparations have been monitored for periods of up to 2 years.

The engraftment of CD34+ cells must be interpreted with the caveat that the durations of the studies to date may be too short to have determined long-term engraftment. In a feline transplant model, exhaustible multipotent progenitors persisted for 1 to 4.5 years.[15,21]

These cells were detectable by fluctuations in the clonal origin of cells contributing to the peripheral blood. It has been speculated that the persistence of such exhaustible multipotent progenitors may increase with the longevity and/or size of the animal. In simplistic terms, the murine and feline model systems suggest that clonal fluctuations might persist for one-tenth to one-third the life span of the animal.[15,17-21] This would suggest that human reconstitution would need to be monitored for at least 7 years posttransplant to establish long-term reconstitution. Thus, there is no firm proof that CD34+ cell preparations contain the true long-term HSC, although the data remains highly suggestive.

The issues surrounding CD34 have recently come to bear on at least 4 independent studies which suggest that, in murine hematopoietic development, long-term reconstituting hematopoietic cells may be CD34 dim/-.[60-63] Most human hematopoietic cells are CD34– and human CD34– cell preparations are not supported in either in vitro or in vivo assays for primitive hematopoietic progenitors. This would suggest that human HSC are CD34+. Alternatively, the assays available for screening hematopoietic progenitors may be artificial environments that simply favor the growth of CD34+ cells. No in vitro culture assay has been clearly demonstrated to support HSC, and these culture systems may support only exhaustible multilineage progenitors.

To isolate CD34– HSC in the absence of an obvious cell surface marker would require that cell populations be selected by a means that does not rely on immunophenotypic markers. Alternative phenotypes for the HSC include a very low incidence for entering the cell cycle and a high degree of resistance to irradiation; however, these are difficult to manipulate for cell isolation strategies.[64,65] One property of HSC that may be used for stem cell isolation purposes is the resistances of HSCs to many cytotoxic drugs that are commonly used in chemotherapy. The mechanisms of resistance seem to be specific for each agent. Some drugs are effluxed from the cell by highly active membrane pumps while others are inactivated by specific cellular enzymes.[60,66,67] These resistance phenotypes have been manipulated for cell isolation by fluorescence activated cell sorting. Murine CD34– HSC have been isolated by selecting cells on the basis of their expression of aldehyde dehydrogenase,[60,66] the enzyme that mediates resistance to cyclophosphamide.[68] Similarly, murine CD34– HSC have been isolated by monitoring dye efflux of the vital DNA stain

Hoechst 33342 and/or the mitochondrial stain Rhodamine-123.[62,69-71] In studies using Hoechst 33342, the fluorescence emission can be visualized in two wavelengths simultaneously to permit the dissection of bone marrow cells into many small subpopulations. One such subfraction is highly enriched for murine CD34– HSC.[62,69]

Our own group has used a dye efflux technique to characterize progenitors within human umbilical cord blood (UCB). The method chosen was one of the strategies used to isolate CD34– HSC from murine bone marrow.[69] This technique relies on the efflux of the vital DNA stain Hoechst 33342, but is probably also dependent upon the condensed chromatin structure of primitive cells. Based on similarities with the fluorescence emission profile of Hoechst-stained murine bone marrow, a dim staining subpopulation (termed the SP) was characterized in human UCB (Storms et al submitted). Initially the CD34– cells within the UCB SP were found to contain many cells obviously committed to the T and/or NK cell lineages. We therefore characterized an SP subpopulation from UCB that was depleted of lineage-committed cells (Lin- UCB). The Lin- UCB SP was comprised nearly equally by CD34+ and CD34– cells. While these percentages fluctuated between UCBs assayed, the cell phenotypes were highly consistent. The CD34+ cells were CD33- CD71- and CD45RA- but were not clearly delineated by their expression of CD38 or CDw90 (Thy-1). All myeloid growth that has been detectable thus far has localized to the CD34+ subfraction of the Lin- UCB SP. The CD34– cells were CD7+ 45RA+ 11b+, but did not express most antigens commonly associated with either the T or NK cell lineages (e.g., CD1a, CD2, CD3, CD4, CD5, CD8, CD56, CDw90). These cells also did not express cell surface antigens commonly associated with activation (e.g., CD38, CD71). We have not been able to culture these CD7+ CD34– Lin- UCB SP cells under any conditions, and therefore we have been unable to assign this cell to any specific hematopoietic lineage.

The Selection of CD34+ Cells

CD34+ cells clearly possess the potential for multilineage development and CD34 may, in fact, define the true HSC. Clinical gene therapy protocols generally use a positive selection strategy for CD34+ cells.[54,56] This may present a second problem in that the crosslinking of the cell surface antigens may provide an inadvertant stimulation that could alter the engraftment potential of the cell. Antigen crosslinking is commonly used to stimulate mitosis in certain cell types, e.g., T cells. No proof exists for any damage sustained by positive selection strategies for CD34+ cells; however, since an absolute purification of HSC is not required it may be advantageous to avoid this issue altogether. Highly enriched populations of progenitor cells can be easily prepared by depleting obvious T cells, B cells, NK cells and monocytes using high gradient magnetic separation.[44,45,72] Lineage-depleted cell preparations that are 50-60% CD34+ are routinely attained from human UCB without positive selection (Storms et al submitted). These cell preparations typically represent only up to about 0.5% of the original white cell content of the UCB and are highly enriched for clonogenic hematopoietic progenitors and for LTC-IC (Storms et al submitted). These cell preparations are enriched enough for gene modification in a clinical setting, have no bias toward a specific stem cell antigen, and have never been stimulated by surface antigen crosslinking.

Gene Delivery into Human Hematopoietic Stem Cells

The Ex Vivo Expansion of HSC

While the positive selection of CD34+ cells may introduce some adverse effect on the outcome of transplants, other factors must be influencing the poor gene delivery into HSC. The preclinical studies optimized conditions for gene transfer into clonogenic progenitor cells and LTC-IC, and these conditions are obviously suboptimal for HSC.[49-53] In these protocols, enriched pools of CD34+ HSC are generally expanded in cytokine cocktails that are known to expand clonogenic progenitors within an LTC-IC fraction of cells. This ex vivo expansion prior to gene transfer is probably the single largest variable to account for a loss of HSC function. Murine HSC have been maintained in short-term ex vivo cultures. In these cultures the HSC compartment is at least partially preserved; however, some loss of HSC is always noted.[31,73] Thus, treating HSC preparations with cytokine cocktails risks the destruction of their potential for long-term engraftment.

The only way to address these concerns would be to more accurately define the conditions for short term culture that leave the HSC compartment most intact. The fundamental question would still remain as to how to assay for human HSC. One means for defining conditions for the ex vivo expansion of HSC might be to assay for the maintenance of SCID mouse repopulating cells (SRC).[30,44,45]

The SRC are more primitive than LTC-IC, although there is no evidence to date that they contain transplantable human HSC. Unfortunately, the SRC assays are expensive and technically demanding. Thus, it would be difficult to rapidly screen a large number of potentially useful conditions for the ex vivo expansion of HSC. Therefore, these assays would be best left as proofs of principle for conditions that were identified in separate in vitro assays.

To date the most stringent gene transfer studies focused on the delivery of genes into LTC-IC. However, the LTC-IC has obviously failed as a readout for gene transfer into HSC. Several lines of evidence now suggest that the traditional LTC-IC, which are expanded on stromal monolayers for 5 weeks, are probably committed progenitors and not HSC. It is now clear that more primitive cells are assayable in vitro. A minor subset of LTC-IC differentiate into assayable clonogenic progenitors only after 10-12 weeks growth on stromal support cultures.[28] These cells have been referred to as extended LTC-IC (eLTC-IC). Gene transfer should be assayable within these primitive subsets of the LTC-IC, and these populations might more accurately reflect gene transfer into HSC.

The eLTC-IC, a 3 month culture system, is nearly as cumbersome as the use of SCID animal models. However, the eLTC-IC may actually be identical to a second primitive subset of LTC-IC that has been referred to as cytokine-resistant cells (CRC). These cells remain dormant for several days after exposure to cytokines, but eventually proceed into the cell cycle. The CRC have been detected using 2 distinct culture systems, and can be assayed within a period of 1-2 weeks.[74,75] Provided that these cells can be shown to be identical to the eLTC-IC, this much shorter culture period would permit a more rapid screening of conditions for the ex vivo culture of HSC.

The CRC phenotype, defined by a resistance to mitotic stimulation, is intriguing in that the HSC rarely divides. In stochastic mathematical models, it has been estimated that feline HSC divide no more than once every 3 weeks.[15] These rare subfractions of LTC-IC may also reconcile the relative success of in vitro gene transfer studies with the failure of the clinical trials for stem cell-based gene therapies. For retrovirus-mediated gene transduction, the cells must proceed into the cell cycle to permit the stable integration of the virus. To date, most gene transfer protocols transduce HSC over a 3 day period of cytokine stimulations. At this timepoint the cytokine-resistant cells are not yet in cycle and would therefore exhibit a low frequency of transduction. At the same time, the cells that are readily stimulated to divide would be transduced with a higher frequency, but are also the cells already committed to differentiation that would be assayable as clonogenic progenitors and as LTC-IC.

Having identified a target cell population that is more primitive than the traditional LTC-IC, it will be important to determine the efficiency of gene delivery into these cells. Recent innovations in gene delivery systems have incorporated the expression of cell surface antigens by the retroviral transducing vector.[76,77] This provides the ability to immediately determine the delivery of foreign genes into specific cells (e.g., CD34+ CD38- cells) by using multiparameter flow cytometry. In studies within our own laboratory, it is evident that when an HSC preparation is placed in culture for gene transduction, the majority of cells that initiate the culture expand rapidly. These cells gradually lose their expression of CD34 and increase in their expression of CD38. A minor subpopulation of cells remain CD34+ CD38- during the 3 day period that the target HSC population is maintained in culture with cytokines. Not surprisingly, the cells that maintain the more primitive phenotype exhibit very low gene transfer.

Conclusions

The prospects for stem cell-based gene therapies for AIDS are promising but clearly challenging. Several potentially useful intracellular inhibitors of HIV replication are now available for testing their true efficacy in a clinical setting. The most fundamental problems faced in this field are those of gene delivery. The central question is how to introduce a gene into a rare, quiescent cell that can not be readily identified by any known phenotype. Yet, even these obstacles are being overcome. The recent description of several assayable cell populations that might contain the HSC (eLTC, cytokine-resistant cells and/or the SCID repopulating cells) will clearly facilitate studies for delivering genes into these rare cells. Furthermore, by using viral vectors that express cell surface markers it is now feasible to accurately, and immediately, assay the delivery of genes into these rare subpopulations.

References

1. Staprans S, Feinberg MB. Natural history and immunopathogenesis of HIV-1 disease. In: Sande MA, Volberding PA, ed. The Medical Management of AIDS. 4th ed. Philadelphia, PA: W.B. Saunders Company, 1995: 38-64.
2. Greene WC. Molecular Insights into HIV-1 infection. In: Sande MA, Volberding PA, ed. The Medical Management of AIDS. 4th ed. Philadelphia, PA: W.B. Saunders Company, 1995: 22-37.
3. Fischl MA. Treatment of HIV infection. In: Sande MA, Volberding PA, ed. The Medical Management of AIDS. Philadelphia, PA: W. B. Saunders Company, 1995: 141-160.
4. Andreoni M, Sarmati L, Ercoli L et al. Correlation between changes in plasma HIV RNA levels and in plasma infectivity in response to antiretroviral therapy. AIDS Res Human Retrovirol 1997; 13:555-561.
5. Hammer SM, Squires KE, Hughes MD et al. A controlled trial of two nucleoside analogs plus indivavir in persons with human immunodeficiency virus infection and CD4 cell counts of 200 per cubic millimeter or less. AIDS Clinical Trials Group 320 Study Team. N Engl J Med 1997; 337:725-733.
6. Baltimore D. Intracellular immunization. Nature 1988;335:395-396.
7. Trono D, Feinberg MB, Baltimore D. HIV-1 gag mutants can dominantly interfere with the replication of the wild-type virus. Cell 1989; 59:113-120.
8. Malim MH, Bohnlein S, Hauber J et al. Functional dissection of the HIV-1 Rev trans-activator—Derivation of a trans-dominant repressor of Rev function. Cell 1989; 58:205-214.
9. Riddell SR, Elliott M, Lewinsohn DA et al. T cell mediated rejection of gene-modified HIV-specific cytotoxic T lymphocytes in HIV-infected patients. Nature Med 1996; 2:165-167.
10. Lee S-W, Gallardo HF, Gaspar O et al. Inhibition of HIV-1 in CEM cells by a potent TAR decoy. Gene Ther 1995; 2:377-384.
11. Lee S-W, Gallardo HF, Gilboa E et al. Inhibition of human immunodeficiency virus type I in human T cells by a potent Rev response element decoy consisting of the 13 nucleotide minimal Rev-binding domain. J Virol 1994; 68:8254-8264.
12. Blaese RM. Progress toward gene therapy. Clin Immunol Immunopath 1991; 61:S47-S55.
13. Ogawa M, Porter PN, Nakahata T. Renewal and commitment to differentiation of hemopoietic stem cells (An interpretative review). Blood 1983; 61:823-829.
14. Lemischka IR. Clonal, in vivo behavior of the totipotent hematopoietic stem cell. Semin Immunol 1991; 3:349-355.
15. Abkowitz JL, Catlin SN, Guttorp P. Evidence that hematopoiesis may be a stochastic process in vivo. Nature Med 1996; 2:190-197.
16. Harrison DE, Astle CM, Lerner C. Number and continuous proliferative pattern of transplanted primitive immunohematopoietic stem cells. Proc Natl Acad Sci USA 1988; 85:822-826.

17. Jordan CT, Lemischka IR. Clonal and systemic analysis of long-term hematopoiesis in the mouse. Genes Devel 1990; 4:220-232.

18. Keller G, Snodgrass R. Life span of multipotential hematopoietic stem cells in vivo. J Exp Med 1990; 171:1407-1418.

19. Snodgrass R, Keller G. Clonal fluctuation within the haematopoietic system of mice reconstituted with retrovirus-infected stem cells. EMBO J 1987; 6:3955-3960.

20. Harrison DE, Zhong R-K. The same exhaustible multilineage precursor produces both myeloid and lymphoid cells as early as 3-4 weeks after marrow transplantation. Proc Natl Acad Sci USA 1992; 89:10134-10138.

21. Abkowitz JL, Persik MT, Shelton GH et al. Behavior of hematopoietic stem cells in a large animal. Proc Natl Acad Sci USA 1995; 92: 2031-2035.

22. Turhan AG, Humphries RK, Phillips GL et al. Clonal hematopoiesis demonstrated by X-linked DNA polymorphisms after allogeneic bone marrow transplantation. N Engl J Med 1989; 320:1655-1661.

23. Nash R, Storb R, Neiman P. Polyclonal reconstitution of human marrow after allogeneic bone marrow transplantation. Blood 1988; 72:2031-2037.

24. Baum CM, Weissman IL, Tsukamoto AS et al. Isolation of a candidate human hematopoietic stem-cell population. Proc Natl Acad Sci USA 1992; 89:2804-2808.

25. Cicuttini FM, Welch K, Boyd AW. Characterization of CD34+HLA-DR-CD38+ and CD34+HLA-DR-CD38- progenitor cells from human umbilical cord blood. Growth Factors 1994; 10:127-34.

26. De Bruyn C, Delforge A, Bron D et al. Comparison of the co-expression of CD38, CD33 and HLA-DR antigens on CD34+ purified cells from human cord blood and bone marrow. Stem Cells 1995; 13:281-288.

27. DiGiusto D, Chen S, Combs J et al. Human fetal bone marrow early progenitors for T, B, and myeloid cells are found exclusively in the population expressing high levels of CD34. Blood 1994; 84:421-432.

28. Hao Q-L, Shah A, Thiemann F et al. A functional comparison of CD34+CD38- cells in cord blood and bone marrow. Blood 1995; 86: 3745-3753.

29. Huang S, Terstappen LWMM. Lymphoid and myeloid differentiation of single human CD34+ HLA-DR+ CD38- hematopoietic stem cells. Blood 1994; 83:1515-1526.

30. Larochelle A, Vormoor J, Hanenberg H et al. Identification of primitive human hematopoietic cells capable of repopulating NOD/SCID mouse bone marrow: Implications for gene therapy. Nature Med 1996; 2:1329-1337.

31. Muench MO, Cupp J, Polakoff J et al. Expression of CD33, CD38, and HLA-DR on CD34+ human fetal liver progenitors with a high proliferative potential. Blood 1994; 83:3170-81.

32. Peault B, Weissman IL, Baum C et al. Lymphoid reconstitution of the human fetal thymus in SCID mice with CD34+ presursor cells. J Exp Med 1991; 174:1283-1286.

33. Thoma SJ, Lamping CP, Ziegler B. Phenotype analysis of hematopoietic CD34+ cell populations derived from human umbilical cord blood using flow cytometry and cDNA-polymerase chain reaction. Blood 1994; 83:2103-2114.

34. Terstappen L, Huang S, Safford M et al. Sequential generations of hematopoietic colonies derived from single nonlineage-committed CD34+CD38- progenitor cells. Blood 1991; 77:1218-1227.

35. Wagner J, Collins D, Fuller S et al. Isolation of small, primitive human hematopoietic stem cells: Distribution of cell surface cytokine receptors and growth in SCID-Hu mice. Blood 1995; 86:512-523.

36. Zanjani ED, Flake AW, Rice H et al. Long-term repopulating ability of xenogeneic transplanted human fetal liver hematopoietic stem cells in sheep. J Clin Invest 1994; 93:1051-1055.

37. Bradley TR, Metcalf D. The growth of mouse bone marrow cells in vitro. Aust J Exp Biol Med Sci 1966; 44:287-292.

38. Dexter TM, Allen TD, Lajtha LG. Conditions controlling the proliferation of haeomatopoietic stem cells in vitro. J Cell Physiol 1977; 91:335-345.

39. Andrews RG, Singer JW, Bernstein ID. Human hematopoietic precursors in long term culture: single CD34+ cells that lack detectable T cell, B cell and myeloid antigens produce multiple multiple colony forming cells when cultured with marrow stromal cells. J Exp Med 1990; 172:355-358.

40. Sutherland H, Eaves C, Eaves A et al. Characterization and partial purification of human marrow cells capable of initiating long-term hematopoiesis in vitro. Blood 1989; 74:1563-1570.

41. Koller MR, Emerson SG, Palsson BO. Large-scale expansion of human stem and progenitor cells from bone marrow mononuclear cells in continuous perfusion cultures. Blood 1993; 82:378-384.

42. Emerson S. Ex vivo expansion of hematopoietic precursors, progenitors, and stem cells: the next generation of cellular therapeutics. Blood 1996; 87:3082-3088.

43. Dick JE. Normal and leukemic human stem cells assayed in SCID mice. Semin Immunol 1996; 8:197-206.

44. Bhatia M, Bonnet D, Kapp U et al. Quantitative analysis reveals expansion of human hematopoietic repopulating cells after short-term ex vivo culture. J Exp Med 1997; 186:619-624.

45. Conneally E, Cashman J, Petzer A et al. Expansion in vitro of transplantable human cord blood stem cells demonstrated using a quantitative assay of their lympho-myeloid repopulating activity in nonobese diabetic-scid/scid mice. Proc Natl Acad Sci USA 1997; 94:9836-9841.

46. Licht T, Aksentijevich I, Gottesman MM et al. Efficient expression of functional human MDR1 gene in murine bone marrow after retroviral transduction of purified hematopoietic stem cells. Blood 1995; 86:111-121.
47. Capel B, Hawley R, Covarrubias L et al. Clonal contributions of small numbers of retrovirally marked hematopoietic stem cells engrafted in unirradiated neonatal W/Wv mice. Proc Natl Acad Sci USA 1989; 86:4564-4568.
48. Lemischka IR, Raulet DH, Mulligan RC. Developmental potential and dynamic behavior of hematopoietic stem cells. Cell 1986; 45:917-927.
49. Hughes PFD, Eaves CJ, Hogge DE et al. High efficiency gene transfer to human hematopoietic cells maintained in long-term marrow culture. Blood 1989; 74:1915-1922.
50. Hughes PFD, Thacker JD, Hogge D et al. Retroviral gene transfer to primitive normal and leukemic hematopoietic cells using clinically applicable procedures. J Clin Invest 1992; 89:1817-1824.
51. Cournoyer D, Scarpa M, Mitani K et al. Gene transfer of adenosine deaminase into primitive human hematopoietic progenitor cells. Hum Gene Ther 1991; 2:203-213.
52. Moritz T, Patel VP, Williams DA. Bone marrow extracellular matrix molecules improve gene transfer into human hematopoietic cells via retroviral vectors. J Clin Invest 1994; 93:1451-1457.
53. Nolta JA, Kohn DB. Comparison of the effects of growth factors on retroviral vector-mediated gene transfer and the proliferative status of human hematopoietic progenitor cells. Human Gene Therapy 1990; 1:257-268.
54. Andrews RG, M BE, Bartelmez SH et al. CD34+ marrow cells, devoid of T and B lymphocytes, reconstitute stable lymphopoiesis and myelopoiesis in lethally irradiated allogeneic baboons. Blood 1992; 80:1693-1701.
55. Bodine DM, Moritz T, Donahue RE et al. Long-term in vivo expression of a murine adenosine deaminase gene in rhesus monkey hematopoietic cells of multiple lineages after retroviral mediated gene transfer into CD34+ bone marrow cells. Blood 1993; 82:1975-1980.
56. Dunbar CE, Cottler-Fox M, O'Shaughnessy JA et al. Retrovirally marked CD34-enriched peripheral blood and bone marrow cells contribute to long-term engraftment after autologous transplantation. Blood 1995; 85:3084-3057.
57. van Beusechem VW, Kukler A, Heidt PJ et al. Long-term expression of human adenosine deaminase in rhesus monkeys transplanted with retrovirus-infected bone-marrow cells. Proc Natl Acad Sci USA 1992; 89:7640-7644.
58. Tjonnfjord GE, Steen R, Veiby OP et al. Evidence for engraftment of donor-type multipotent CD34+ cells in a patient with selective T lymphocyte reconstitution after bone marrow transplantation for B-SCID. Blood 1994; 84:3584-3589.

59. Berenson RJ, Bensinger WI, Hill RS et al. Engraftment after infusion of CD34+ marrow cells in patients with breast cancer or neuroblastoma. Blood 1991; 77:1717-1722.

60. Jones RJ, Collector MI, Barber JP et al. Characterization of mouse lymphohematopoietic stem cells lacking spleen colony-forming activity. Blood 1996; 88:487-491.

61. Osawa M, Hanada K-I, Hamada H et al. Long-term reconstitution by a single CD34-low/negative hematopoietic stem cell. Science 1996; 273:242-245.

62. Goodell MA, Rosenzweig M, Kim H et al. Dye efflux studies suggest the existence of CD34-negative/low hematopoietic stem cells in multiple species. Nature Med 1997; 3:1337-1345.

63. Morel F, Galy A, Chen B et al. Characterization of CD34 negative hematopoietic stem cells in murine bone marrow. Blood 1996; 88 (supplement 1):629a.

64. Fleming WH, Alpern EJ, Uchida N et al. Functional heterogeneity is associated with the cell cycle status of murine hematopoietic stem cells. J Cell Biol 1993; 122:897-902.

65. Ploemacher RE, van Os R, van Beurden CAJ et al. Murine haemopoietic stem cells with long-term engraftment and marrow repopulating ability are more resistant to gamma-irradiation than are spleen colony forming cells. Int J Radiat Biol 1992; 61:489-499.

66. Jones RJ, Barber JP, Vala MS et al. Assessment of aldehyde dehydrogenase in viable cells. Blood 1995; 85:2742-2748.

67. Chaudhary PM, Roninson IB. Expression and activity of p-glycoprotein, a multidrug efflux pump, in human hematopoietic stem cells. Cell 1991; 66:85-94.

68. Hilton J. Role of aldehyde dehydrogenase in cyclophosphamide-resistant L1210 leukemia. Cancer Res 1984; 44:5156-5160.

69. Goodell M, Brose K, Paradis G et al. Isolation and functional properties of murine hematopoietic stem cells that are replicating in vivo. J Exp Med 1996; 183:1797-1806.

70. Wolf NS, Kone A, Priestley GV, et al. In vivo and in vitro characterization of long-term repopulating primitive hematopoietic cells isolated by sequential Hoechst 33342-rhodamine 123 FACS selection. Exp Hematol 1993; 21:614-622.

71. Li CL, Johnson GR. Rhodamine123 reveals heterogenity within murine lin-, Sca-1+ hemopoietic stem cells. J Exp Med 1992; 175: 1443-1447.

72. Thomas TE, Abraham SJR, Otter AJ et al. High gradient magnetic separation of cells on the basis of expression levels of cell surface antigens. J Immunol Methods 1992; 154:245-252.

73. van der Loo JCM, Ploemacher RE. Marrow- and spleen-seeding efficiencies of all murine hematopoietic stem cell subsets are decreased by preincubation with hematopoietic growth factors. Blood 1995; 85:2598-2606.

74. Traycoff CM, Kosak ST, Grigsby S et al. Evaluation of ex vivo expansion potential of cord blood and bone marrow hemaotpoietic progenitor cells using cell tracking and limiting dilution analysis. Blood 1995; 85:2059-2068.

75. Ponchio L, Conneally E, Eaves C. Quantitation of the quiescent fraction of long-term culture-initiating cells in normal human blood and marrow and the kinetics of their growth factor-stimulated entry into S-phase in vitro. Blood 1995; 86:3314-3321.

76. Phillips K, Gentry T, McCowage G et al. Cell-surface markers for assessing gene transfer into human hematopoietic cells. Nature Med 1996; 2:1154-1156.

77. McCowage GB, Phillips KL, Gentry TL et al. Multiparameter fluorescence activated cell sorting analysis of retroviral vector gene transfer into primitive umbilical cord blood cells. Exp Hematol 1998; 26:288-298.

CHAPTER 7

Animal Models of Gene Therapy for AIDS

Linda M. Kofeldt and David Camerini

Introduction

An appropriate test system for AIDS gene therapies must possess several features. It must readily allow the introduction of gene therapeutics to be tested and must reproduce, at least in part, the pathogenesis of HIV-1 in infected people. The value of animal models for testing anti-HIV-1 gene therapy is clear from the inadequacy of tissue culture systems in reproducing the pathogenesis of patient derived strains of HIV-1. T lymphoblastoid cell lines (T-LCL) are not permissive for most clinical isolates of HIV-1 since they lack CCR5,[1] and primary T cells are difficult to maintain for long periods without compromising their diversity. Furthermore, in tissue culture four of the nine genes of HIV-1 are dispensable for replication,[2] while in pathogenic infections in humans, all nine genes are universally maintained.[3] These deficiencies have led to the use of several animal models for the study of HIV-1 pathogenesis. Several model systems use immunodeficient mice engrafted with human immune cells while other models use one of several species of macaque infected with SIV, a virus which is highly related to HIV-2 and more distantly related to HIV-1.[4] Some of these animal models of HIV and SIV pathogenesis have been modified to allow the testing of potential gene therapeutic agents for human and simian AIDS.

Gene Therapy for HIV Infection, edited by Clay Smith. © 1998 Springer-Verlag and R.G. Landes Company.

SCID Mice

A mouse with severe combined immune deficiency (SCID) was discovered by Bosma in 1983, and the defect was shown to be caused by a new recessive mutation.[5] SCID mice have a near total absence of normal B and T cells but possess normal NK cell function. They have been used as models to study lymphocyte subsets in healthy and diseased human donors. SCID mice were also shown to be permissive recipients of human hemopoietic cells. Currently, two model systems which employ SCID mice are in use to study HIV-1 pathogenesis: the human peripheral blood lymphocyte SCID (hu-PBL-SCID) mouse developed by Mosier and colleagues,[6] and the SCID-human thymus/liver (SCID-hu) mouse developed by McCune, Weissman and colleagues.[7]

The hu-PBL-SCID Mouse

In this model, hu-PBL are injected intraperitoneally into SCID mice. This leads to the selective survival and expansion of human $CD3^+$ T cells; smaller numbers of human B cells, monocytes, and NK cells also survive.[8,9] Human cells can be recovered from the spleen, bone marrow, and lymph nodes that drain the peritoneal cavity as well as from the site of injection. In addition, small numbers of human T cells can be recovered from peripheral blood and other lymph nodes of the hu-PBL-SCID mouse model.[8] Mosier and others have shown that human T cells in this model can be infected in vivo with HIV-1 with subsequent loss of $CD4^+$ T cells.[10,11] Nonsyncytium inducing HIV-1 isolates, however, are more pathogenic in this model, while they are not associated with acute pathogenesis in infected people.[12,13] This model has been used to show that anti-retroviral treatment of SCID mice containing hu-PBL from HIV-1-infected individuals inhibited HIV-1 replication and the loss of human $CD4^+$ cells,[11] and to assess the efficacy of vaccines to HIV-1.[14] Since the hu-PBL-SCID model utilizes differentiated hemopoietic cells as opposed to hemopoietic stem cells, it is not an ideal model for long lasting multilineage gene therapy, which may be required for effective AIDS gene therapy. A therapy relying on the transduction of mature T cells would likely require repeated treatments to be effective and would not provide protection against infection of macrophages by HIV-1.[15] Nevertheless, transduced PBMC could be injected into SCID mice and challenged with HIV-1; however, this has not yet been done.

The SCID-hu Mouse

The SCID-hu mouse was conceived by McCune et al in an effort to provide a suitable small animal model for the study of the pathogenesis and treatment of AIDS.[16] The model was initially created by surgical implantation of human fetal thymus fragments under the renal capsule of a C.B-17 *scid/scid* mouse. This permitted growth of the thymic fragments and differentiation of the progenitor cells, but both were transient. Subsequent SCID-hu models utilized both human fetal thymus and human fetal liver implanted under the renal capsule of the SCID mouse.[7] In this model, the implanted human tissue forms a conjoined organ which provides a suitable microenvironment for the differentiation of human hemopoietic precursor cells into thymocytes and mature T cells. This conjoint organ was a distinct improvement over implanted fetal thymus alone; large implants with ongoing thymopoiesis were observed over a period of up to 12 months in over 80% of the grafts.[17] Thymus/liver grafts display the architecture of the normal human thymus with intervening islets of liver which continually provide precursor cells. The SCID-hu graft becomes populated with thymocyte subsets similar to that of the normal human thymus, containing $CD4^- CD8^-$ stage I thymocytes, $CD4^+ CD8^+$ stage II thymocytes and both $CD4^+$ and $CD8^+$ mature stage III cells. Thymocytes proliferate during stage II, so $CD4^+ CD8^+$ double positive cells constitute 70% to 90% of the thymocytes.

When infected with HIV-1, the human $CD4^+$ cells, both single and double positive, are susceptible to HIV-1 infection and pathogenesis.[18,19,20] This pathogenesis is dependent upon *nef* gene function,[21] as is HIV-1 pathogenesis in infected people.[22] Studies in our laboratory and by others have shown that nonsyncytium inducing (NSI) HIV-1 isolates from asymptomatic individuals are weakly pathogenic in the SCID-hu mouse, but syncytium inducing (SI) isolates taken from these same individuals at later stages of infection, i.e., obtained at the onset of rapid $CD4^+$ cell depletion, are cytopathic in the SCID-hu mouse. (Camerini D, Connor R, Zack J et al manuscript submitted).[23] Therefore, the SCID-hu mouse model accurately reflects this aspect of the diverse pathogenicity of patient isolates of HIV-1, making it an attractive model system.

Akkina et al first demonstrated that SCID-hu mice can be irradiated, with resultant destruction of human thymocytes, without disruption of the thymopoietic environment of the graft.[24] The thymus/liver graft can then be repopulated with human thymocytes derived from retroviral vector transformed $CD34^+$ precursor cells obtained from human fetal liver, bone marrow or human umbilical cord blood. In 1994, Akkina et al transduced $CD34^+$ hemopoietic progenitor cells in vitro with an amphotropic. Moloney murine leukemia virus (MMLV)-based retrovirus vector carrying the neomycin phosphotransferase gene (*npt*) and injected the transduced cells directly into the thymus/liver implants of SCID-hu mice following sublethal irradiation. Human Y chromosome-specific PCR was used to distinguish previously engrafted fetal thymus/liver cells (female) from progeny of the repopulating $CD34^+$ cells derived from human fetal liver (male). Each of the irradiated mice which received transduced $CD34^+$ cells showed normal distribution profiles of $CD4^+$ $CD8^+$ immature cells and both $CD4^+$ $CD8^-$ and $CD4^-$ $CD8^+$ mature human thymocytes, indicating reconstitution of the thymocyte compartment from the transduced $CD34^+$ cells. It was determined that 5 x 10^4 $CD34^+$ cells are required to reconstitute a thymic implant with cells containing the transduced vector. If approximately 0.1% to 1.0% of $CD34^+$ cells constitute true pluripotent stem cells,[25] it would appear that 50 to 500 stem cells are required for reconstitution in this system, although more mature thymocyte precursors could be responsible for the thymocyte repopulation seen in these experiments. There was no apparent deleterious effect on thymocyte differentiation due to transduction. Three percent of the thymocytes contained *npt* vector sequences with *npt* mRNA expressed at low levels, detectable by RT PCR with ^{32}P labeled primers. These experiments established the SCID-hu mouse as an ideal system in which to test anti-HIV-1 gene therapies based on transduction of primitive thymocyte precursors or multipotent hemopoietic stem cells and subsequent assay of their efficacy in protecting thymocytes from HIV-1.

We have transduced $CD34^+$ cells with the retroviral vector MN (provided by Drs. Clay Smith and Eli Gilboa of Duke University), which encodes the human nerve growth factor receptor (NGFR), as a marker gene. In vitro, NGFR was expressed on 30% of the $CD34^+$ cells 3 days post infection (data not shown). These cells were then injected into SCID-hu mice following irradiation with 400 cGy from a $^{137}Cesium$ source. Two of four injected mice, biopsied 5 weeks post injection expressed NGFR on 7% and 16% of the thymocytes respectively (Fig 7.1). At week nine, one remaining live mouse expressed NGFR on greater than 22% of the thymocytes (Fig. 7.2). A normal distribution of thymocyte subsets was observed in the mice which received transduced cells, indicating that the transgene and vector sequences had no deleterious effects on thymocyte development. Control mice implanted with tissue from the same donor and irradiated in the same manner but not injected with transduced hemopoietic precursor cells had no thymocytes at biopsy. Our results show the utility of surface markers for detecting transduced cells in this system and the value of human fetal liver as a source of transducible thymocyte precursors. A surface marker allows flow cytometric detection of transduced cells as well as purification of transduced cells by FACS or other means. Additionally, our results with fetal liver derived CD34+ cells suggest that these cells are readily transduced with murine retroviral vectors.

A variation of the SCID-hu model was utilized by Champseix and colleagues.[26] CD34$^+$ cells from human umbilical cord blood were cocultured with CRIP MFG-mouse CD2 (mCD2) cells that produce murine retroviral vectors encoding the mCD2 antigen, a cell surface glycoprotein. Human fetal thymus fragments were dissected and depleted of endogenous thymocytes by organ culture at 24°C for 3 to 5 days. Some thymus fragments were irradiated at a single dose of 250 cGy. The fragments were then injected with 2 x 10^4 transduced CD34$^+$ cells and inserted under the renal capsule of SCID mice. Implants were biopsied from 5 to 10 weeks post engraftment and thymocyte subsets were in normal distribution for the duration of engraftment. Four of nine experimental mice expressed mCD2, ranging from 5 to 9% of total cells in thymus grafts. This system, while likely to give smaller grafts and fewer transduced thymocytes than the model developed by Akkina and colleagues, may have a lower background of untransduced cells.

Recently, Chen, Zack and colleagues described the use of a cell surface reporter gene, mouse *thy-1.2*, in their AIDS gene therapy model system.[27] They transduced human CD34$^+$ cells with a murine retroviral vector bearing the *thy-1.2* marker and pseudotyped with vesicular stomatitis virus G protein. The cell population was further enriched for CD34$^+$ cells expressing Thy-1.2 by FACS, then injected into thymus/liver grafts of sublethally irradiated SCID-hu mice. Reconstitution of the thymus/liver graft with the selected cells resulted in normal distribution of thymocyte subsets. The proportion of cells expressing Thy-1.2 in unsorted thymocytes was 21%; sorting increased Thy-1.2 expression to greater than 80%, with 98%

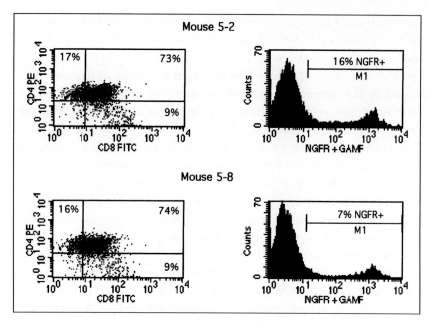

Fig. 7.1. CD4 vs. CD8 and NGFR expression on thymocytes derived from MFG-NGFR transformed CD34+ hemopoietic precursor cells in irradiated SCID-hu mice. Mice were biopsised 5 weeks post introduction of transduced precursor cells and the cells were stained with CD4-PE and CD8-FITC and separately with anti-NGFR mAb followed by goat anti-mouse IgG conjugated to FITC (GAMF).

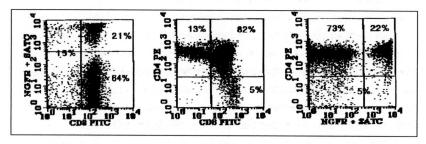

Fig. 7.2. NGFR vs. CD8, CD4 vs. NGFR expression on thymocytes derived from MFG-NGFR transformed CD34+ hemopoietic precursor cells 9 weeks post introduction into irradiated SCID-hu mouse 5-2. Cells were stained with CDr-PE, CD8-FITC and anti-NGFR-biotin mAbs followed by streptavidin conjugated to Tricolor (SATC).

expression observed in one animal. Thy-1.2 was expressed equally in all thymocyte subsets, indicating expression of the vector throughout the process of differentiation. These results illustrate the use of cell surface marker transduced cells purified by FACS in repopulating the thymocyte compartment of SCID-hu mice. This system allows the investigator to obtain a very high proportion of transduced thymocytes which may be required to effectively test AIDS gene therapeutic agents in this model system.

The first test of a gene therapeutic against HIV-1 infection in T cells derived from transduced hemopoietic stem cells was reported by Bonyhadi et al.[28] Previous in vitro studies had shown that a transdominant negative mutant form of HIV-1 Rev, RevM10, was able to inhibit HIV-1 replication in the CEM T-LCL and in primary T cells following MMLV vector-mediated transfer of the RevM10-encoding gene into target cells.[29,30] Bonyhadi and colleagues used an MMLV-based retroviral vector which coexpressed RevM10 and mouse CD8-α chain, from a single mRNA using an internal ribosome entry site (IRES). Mouse CD8 (mCD8) expression was used as an indicator of RevM10 protein expression. The control population of cells was transduced with a vector which coexpressed a noncoding mutated *RevM10* gene (ΔM10) with mCD8. Human umbilical cord blood and granulocyte colony-stimulating factor (G-CSF) mobilized peripheral blood cells were enriched by positive selection with mAbs against surface CD34, transduced with either vector, and stained for cell surface markers. The mCD8 marker was expressed on 8-35% of the CD34$^+$ cells; these cells were sorted to achieve 59-93% purity and were injected into the thymus/liver grafts of SCID-hu mice. At 7 to 9 weeks postinjection, the grafts were removed and partial reconstitution of the grafts with donor cells was observed, with a normal distribution of thymocyte subsets. Surface mCD8 was expressed in approximately 18% of the reconstituted cells derived from mobilized peripheral blood cells and in 10 to 50% of reconstituted cells derived from human umbilical cord blood. These thymocytes were stimulated with PHA and expanded in tissue culture, then infected with the molecular clone HIV-1-JR-CSF at an MOI of 2 x 10^{-2} or with the clinical isolate EW at an MOI of 4 to 8 x 10^{-3}. Virus replication in control thymocytes produced a 3 order of magnitude increase in p24 production at 5 days, while p24 levels in RevM10 producing cells were too low to measure by p24 ELISA in JR-CSF infected cells. In cells infected with the patient isolate EW, RevM10 conferred some protection against HIV-1 replication, with a reduction of almost 2 orders of magnitude in the RevM10 expressing cells as compared to control at 5 days post infection.[28] While these results are quite encouraging, it should be noted that transduced cells were challenged in vitro rather than in SCID-hu mice because the vectors used did not express the mCD8 marker well in vivo. Therefore, although the SCID-hu system was used to allow efficient development of thymocytes from transduced precursor cells, its power as a model of HIV-1 mediated pathogenesis in the thymus was not exploited.

The SCID-hu Bone Model

Although the SCID-hu thymus/liver mouse model provides a good model of human thymopoiesis, evaluation of myeloid and B cell progeny of hemopoietic stem cells is better studied in the context of the bone marrow. The SCID-hu bone model was developed by Kyoizumi, McCune and colleagues by subcutaneous implantation of normal human fetal bone into the SCID mouse.[31] At 4 to 6 weeks post procedure, these implants were vascularized and histologically similar to normal human fetal bone marrow. At 20 weeks post implantation, proliferation and differentiation of human hemopoietic cells was maintained in over 90% of the grafts. Additional studies showed that human hemopoietic progenitor cells from fetal human bone implanted into SCID mice retained multilineage potential and were capable of repopulation of both lymphoid and myeloid cells following secondary transfer into SCID-hu thymus/liver mice or SCID-hu bone mice.[32] Su, Kaneshima and colleagues have used the SCID-hu bone model to show inhibition of HIV-1 replication in vitro in monocytes/macrophages derived from transduced hemopoietic stem cells which express RevM10.[33] Human umbilical cord blood was the source of CD34[+] cells which were transduced with the retroviral vector coexpressing RevM10 and mCD8. Expression of mCD8 was seen in up to 29% of transduced cells. The cells were then injected into sublethally irradiated SCID-hu bone mice. There was efficient reconstitution of the human bone marrow, verified by HLA typing, and expression of the mCD8 gene in up to 54% of the reconstituted cells at 8 weeks post injection. Like the work of Bonyhadi et al,[28] this system shows promise as a model of AIDS gene therapy in mononuclear phagocytes, but the full potential of the system has yet to be exploited, since the cells were challenged with HIV-1 in vitro. Furthermore, if this model were combined with the SCID-hu thymus/

liver model and both grafts were repopulated from a single pool of transduced precursor cells, multilineage AIDS gene therapy could be tested.

Bone Marrow SCID-hu Mice

During the same year that the hu-PBL-SCID and SCID-hu thymus/liver models were reported, another system to repopulate immune-deficient mice with human hemopoietic stem cells was described by John Dick and colleagues.[34] They intravenously injected 10^7 human bone marrow cells into sublethally irradiated CBA/J and *bg/nu/xid* mice. After 14 days, human DNA was detected in the bone marrow and spleen of *bg/nu/xid* mice; in vitro colony-forming assays of single cell suspensions of bone marrow and spleen demonstrated the presence of a population of human progenitor cells which produced colonies viable for greater than 12 days in culture. Later work by this group showed that human bone marrow cells engrafted to higher levels in SCID mice as compared to *bg/nu/xid* mice, and they have continued to use this model to study human hemopoietic stem cells.[35]

Goldstein and colleagues have successfully used the model first described by Dick and colleagues to attain engraftment of both human lymphoid and myeloid lineages within the SCID mouse bone marrow.[36] They injected SCID mice with human fetal bone marrow cells (BM-SCID-hu) or human fetal liver cells (Liv-SCID-hu) to engraft mouse bone marrow.[37] SCID mice were injected in the tail vein with 4×10^7 cultured human fetal bone marrow or human fetal liver cells. At 4 months post transplant, the Liv-SCID-hu mice were sacrificed, and the mouse bone marrow showed the presence of human hemopoietic cells of both lymphoid and myeloid lineages, showing that the cultured fetal liver cells could engraft SCID mice in the absence of exogenous human cytokines. Mouse bone marrow was evaluated at 7 to 8 months after transplant and showed the presence of human $CD34^+$ precursor cells and immature $CD10^+$, $CD20^-$ B cells. Human $CD45^+$ cells were detected in the peripheral blood of 100% of the BM-SCID-hu mice at 3 months and 75% of these mice at 6 months post-transplant. Irradiated SCID mice were then injected with human fetal bone marrow cells or human fetal liver cells transduced with retroviral vectors bearing the *npt* gene. One month post-transplantation, retroviral sequences were present in the peripheral blood mononuclear cells in 57% (8/14) of the animals examined.

Mouse bone marrow was examined from 3 to 7 months post transplantation and the retroviral vector was seen in up to 30% of the human colony forming units (CFU) present. Examination of peripheral blood at the same time showed a population of human $CD45^+$ cells, ranging from 1 to 38% of the total cells. The retroviral vector borne *npt* gene was detected in 5 of 11 mice at 3 to 7 months post implantation. Since no T cells were seen in the peripheral blood of these mice due to the absence of a human thymic microenvironment, they next implanted human fetal thymus into six SCID mice previously injected with human fetal bone marrow or liver cells. Three months post implantation, these mice had an average of 21% human $CD45^+$, 12% human $CD4^+$ and 3% human $CD8^+$ cells in their peripheral blood. Three SCID mice were implanted with human fetal thymus as well as bone marrow cells transduced with the MMLV based vector My-2, pseudotyped with GALV *env* by the PG13 packaging cell line. Three months post transplant, the retroviral vector was detected by PCR in the bone marrow and immature $CD4^+$ $CD8^+$ thymocytes from the grafts of two mice and in $CD4^+$ $CD8^-$ cells in the peripheral blood and thymic implant of another BM-thy-SCID-hu mouse. The SCID mouse peripheral blood engraftment with human leukocytes obtained by these investigators is particularly impressive; it is not clear why this system works better than the SCID-hu thymus/liver mouse in this regard. These investigators, however, have yet to achieve high levels of gene transfer in their system.

Strengths and Weaknesses of the SCID Mouse Models

Despite their advantages, none of the SCID mouse models described above are representative of all aspects of HIV-1 pathogenesis in humans. The thy/liv SCID-hu seems to be an accurate model of infection of the human thymus but not the entire human immune system. The hu-PBL-SCID mouse may be a good model of the establishment of infection in a naive host but it clearly does not reflect later events in the course of a human infection. The BM-SCID-thy and Liv-SCID-thy models show promise in reconstituting lymphoid organs as well as peripheral blood. None of the other mouse models contain many human T cells and therefore can only model the infection of mononuclear phagocytes. In the future, the use of more completely immunodeficient mice may make it possible to more fully establish a human immune system in the SCID mouse. This would provide a better model of HIV-1 pathogenesis and AIDS gene therapy.

In spite of its limitations, the SCID-hu mouse remains the most useful small animal model for further preclinical evaluation of retroviral mediated gene transfer into human hemopoietic stem cells and evaluation of AIDS gene therapies.

While depletion of $CD4^+$ cells is the end effect of infection with HIV-1, the mechanism or mechanisms of cell death in AIDS has remained unclear. Various mechanisms have been proposed including apoptosis,[38,39] immune-mediated lysis,[40,41] single-cell lysis,[42] and syncytia formation.[43] There are no conclusive data demonstrating the mechanism of cell death in people infected with HIV-1. In the SCID-hu model, however, both apoptosis[20,44] and direct killing of infected lymphocytes have been reported.[45] An understanding of the mechanism or mechanisms of cell death in HIV-1 infection may be crucial in designing gene therapeutics for AIDS, as it would indicate which population of cells requires protection—infected cells only or all cells bearing certain receptors such as CD4. Studies in the various SCID mouse model systems may help resolve these issues, since many manipulations can be done which would be impossible in patients.

Primate Models

The close genetic relationship of humans to apes and monkeys makes these animals relevant models for preclinical study of gene therapy for AIDS. However, the study of HIV-1 pathogenesis in a primate model has been hindered by the lack of disease production following inoculation with HIV-1 in nonhuman primate species. Chimpanzees (*Pan troglodytes*) were the first primates in which infection following injection with HIV-1 was established, but there has been little or no progression to AIDS.[46,47] Pigtailed macaques (*Macaca nemestrina*) were inoculated with HIV-1 and seroconverted by 4 weeks post inoculation.[48] HIV-1 specific DNA was present in PBMC for up to 52 weeks and there was persistent antibody response. The macaques showed transient lymphadenopathy after inoculation, but no lasting evidence of disease. $CD4^+$ T cell counts remained normal at 80 weeks post inoculation. Infection of macaques with SIV causes a fatal disease whose pathogenesis is similar to HIV-1 infection in humans.[49] This is the best available primate model for the study of AIDS pathogenesis. Since nonhuman primates have also been used in studies of hemopoietic stem cell gene transfer and transplantation, the basis of a model for AIDS gene therapy exists using

SIV and rhesus (*Macaca mulatta*) or other macaque species. This system, which has yet to be fully exploited, is potentially very powerful but is limited by the use of SIV instead of HIV-1.

Gene Transfer into Primate Hemopoietic Precursor Cells

There is a considerable body of literature on bone marrow gene transfer in nonhuman primates, since monkeys, especially macaques, have been used extensively for investigations of bone marrow transplantation (BMT).[50,51] In the first reported bone marrow cell (BMC) gene transfer study in monkeys, three murine retroviral vectors based on Moloney murine leukemia virus (MMLV) were used.[52,53,54] The best results were seen with SAX, an N2 based vector, containing the *npt* gene, with an SV40 promoter-driven human adenosine deaminase (ADA) gene downstream of *npt*. Of 8 cynomolgus monkeys (*Macaca fascicularis*) subjected to irradiation and autologous BMT with transduced cells, 5 showed leukocyte reconstitution. In four of the reconstituted animals, human ADA enzymatic activity could be detected, albeit at very low levels. Bodine and colleagues transduced 3 rhesus monkey bone marrow aspirates with N263A2 cells, a high titer amphotropic vector producing cell line which also secretes gibbon IL-3 and human IL-6.[55] The animals were reinfused with their transduced autologous bone marrow and all 3 were positive for N2 provirus from day 20 to day 99 post transplant (end of follow-up).

The retrovirus producer cell line POC-1, containing the retroviral vector LgAL, was used by van Beusechem and colleagues to transduce rhesus BMC.[56] The vector expressed the human ADA gene under the control of a hybrid LTR, with enhancer sequences of the polyoma virus mutant F101 replacing those of MMLV. They cocultured rhesus BMC with POC-1 cells in the presence of 3 different concentrations of hemopoietic growth factors: IL-3 at the lowest concentration necessary to promote CFU-C formation, or minimal IL-3 supplemented with IL-1 alpha, or excess IL-3. Irradiated animals whose cells had been exposed to IL-1 alpha showed persistent provirus for only 112 days, and the provirus was seen almost exclusively in PBMC, indicating that only committed progenitor cells were transduced. Conversely, irradiated animals whose cells were not exposed to IL-1α showed low levels of transduction of pluripotent hemopoietic stem cells (PHSC) as evidenced by detection of provirus in 0.01 to 0.1% of PBMC for more than 2 years and in the same percentage of granulocytes for more than one year post-transplant.

Andrews and colleagues showed that CD34$^+$ cells of baboons have multilineage repopulating capabilities in vivo.[57] Many investigators utilized CD34$^+$ subpopulations of BMC for transduction to increase the number of transduced PHSC. Efficient transduction of rhesus CD34$^+$ cells without coculture with stroma or producer cells was demonstrated by Xu and colleagues.[58] They harvested BMC from rhesus monkeys, purified CD34$^+$ cells and transduced them with fresh supernatant with a retroviral vector titer of 10^8/ml. The vector used was LG, a MMLV-based vector which includes the glucocerebrosidase (GC) cDNA driven by the MMLV LTR. The BMC were re-transduced daily with fresh supernatant for four days prior to autologous transplantation into irradiated monkeys (650 Rads). In three animals, they found GC DNA sequences by quantitative PCR in 1 to 14% of peripheral blood B cells 15 to 18 months post-BMT. Gene transfer was achieved in 5 to 16% of BMC and 12 to 22% of popliteal lymph node cells in these animals at 20 months postinfusion.

Kaptein and colleagues reported persistence of retroviral vector transduced cells three years post-transplant of transduced CD34$^+$ BMC.[59] They used the recombinant retroviral vector-producing cell line CRIP/MFG-ADA which, like the POC-1 producer cell line previously used by this group, is derived from a CRIP packaging cell line. The differences in the two lines include the vectors used and the fact that CRIP/MFG-ADA produces a vector titer approximately 25-fold higher than that of POC-1. BMC from two rhesus monkeys were enriched for CD34$^+$ cells, then cocultured on irradiated CRIP/MFG-ADA cells in the presence of rhesus IL-3, then autologously transplanted. To measure initial transduction efficiency, the cells were plated on media selective for ADA overexpression. In vitro transduction efficiency was 66% and 40% respectively for the two monkeys; this was a significant improvement over that seen with POC-1 under the same conditions, 4% and 20% respectively.[60] Following BMT, the hemopoietic systems of both animals regenerated rapidly and were within the normal range for unmanipulated grafts.[61] The animals were followed for one and three years respectively; at the latest time points analyzed, approximately 0.1% of PBMC and 0.01% of granulocytes showed the presence of integrated vector sequences. Semiquantitative PCR analysis was used to compare the monkeys receiving stem cell enriched BMC cocultured with CRIP/MFG-ADA to those receiving BMC cocultured with POC-1. The estimated frequency of PBMC carrying provirus was considerably higher in the

CRIP/MFG-ADA group, but there was no difference in the granulo-cyte transduction efficiency between the two groups. Therefore, while CRIP/MFG-ADA was more efficient in transducing a PBMC precursor, it was not able to improve transduction efficiency of true HSC or granulocyte precursors and in vivo transduction efficiencies following ex vivo gene transfer remained low.

Primate Models for AIDS Gene Therapy

Differentiation of CD4+ T cells is largely restricted to the microenvironment of the thymus, making in vitro analysis of T cells derived from genetically modified CD34+ cells difficult.[62,63] Johnson and colleagues developed an in vitro rhesus thymic stromal culture system that supports T cell differentiation of CD34+ progenitor cells, and have used this system to study T cell differentiation of human and rhesus CD34+ cells.[64] Thymic tissue from fetal rhesus macaques was minced and then digested into a single-cell suspension from which thymic stromal cultures were established. After 7 days of culture, immunohistochemical studies showed a heterogeneous mixture of cells, with fibroblasts, thymic epithelial cells, and macrophages identified. MHC class II staining was seen mainly in the areas where thymic epithelial cells were identified, while MHC class I expression was more uniformly distributed throughout the stromal culture. The thymic stromal cultures were inoculated with purified early progenitor CD34+ CD3− cells derived from either human or macaque bone marrow harvest. Over 21 days, there was a sequential pattern of cell surface marker expression, indicating differentiation in both the macaque and human CD34+ progenitor cells which was consistent with T cell differentiation in fetal thymus.[65,66,67] There was no development of CD3+ lymphocytes in thymic stromal cultures inoculated with rhesus bone marrow depleted of CD34+ cells or in cultures which did not receive CD34+ BMC, indicating that rhesus T lymphocytes arose from the inoculated CD34+ cells and not from the thymic stromal monolayer. Since the human CD3 mAb used for phenotyping did not recognize rhesus T cells, all human T cells arose from the inoculation of human CD34+ cells and not from the rhesus thymic stromal cells.[68] Expression of the recombinase activation gene RAG-2, which is selectively expressed in developing lymphocytes, was detectable in thymic cultures after inoculation with CD34+ cells but not in CD34+ cells prior to culture on the thymic stromal monolayer or in the monolayers alone, providing additional evidence that the

T cells arising in these cultures resulted from in vitro lymphopoiesis. The T cells derived by culture of precursor cells on thymic stroma showed normal phenotypes and responded to mitogenic stimuli. Repeated rounds of stimulation resulted in continued expansion of T cell progeny. Rhesus CD34$^+$ cells cultured on thymic stroma were exposed to SIVmac$_{239}$ at a multiplicity of infection of 0.01 at days 0, 7 and 14 following the initiation of coculture. No SIV replication was seen in CD34$^+$ cells infected on day 0 or in thymic stromal monolayers not inoculated with CD34$^+$ cells. However, rhesus cells infected on days 7 (predominately CD4+ CD8+) and day 14 (CD4+ CD8+, CD4+ CD8-, and CD4-CD8+) were highly permissive to infection with SIVmac$_{239}$ in the absence of mitogenic stimulation. Peak levels of SIV p27 antigen of 23 ng/ml were observed on day 18 following infection.

After showing that rhesus and human CD34$^+$ cells can grow and differentiate on a rhesus thymic stromal monolayer, this group next transduced rhesus CD34$^+$ cells with the LN retroviral vector containing the *npt* gene.[69] Following transduction, cells were cocultured with rhesus thymic stroma for 14 days. The T cell progeny were then stimulated with concanavalin A, irradiated human PBMC, and IL-2, and placed under G418 selection for 28 days. The cells were stained for T cell antigens and sorted to obtain a highly purified CD3$^+$ population. Semiquantitative DNA PCR documented the presence of *npt* DNA in 50 to 100% of the cultured cells, while analysis of *npt* expression by reverse transcriptase PCR showed expression of *npt* at a level comparable to that of a transformed cell line stable transduced with LN.

Recently, Johnson, Lisziewicz and colleagues showed that an antisense *tat* gene in combination with a polymeric TAR sequence (*antitat* gene), inhibited SIV and HIV-1 replication in hemopoietic cells derived from transduced progenitor cells.[70] CD34$^+$ cells were obtained from rhesus bone marrow harvest or human umbilical cord blood. The cells were transduced with a double copy retroviral vector containing the *antitat* gene under control of the HIV-1 LTR and *npt*, or with a control vector containing *npt* alone. As assessed by outgrowth of CFU in the presence of the neomycin analog G418, transduction of CD34$^+$ cells by the vector bearing the *antitat* gene and *npt* resulted in 14 to 30% G418 resistant colonies; similar results were seen with the *npt* control vector. The *antitat* gene was not toxic to the development of hemopoietic lineages, with similar

frequencies of myelomonocytic and erythroid colonies seen as compared to control. In addition, there was normal T cell differentiation
in those CD34$^+$ cells transduced with *antitat*. Transduced CD34$^+$ cells
were cultured on a rhesus thymic stromal monolayer as described
above. Following expansion and restimulation, rhesus CD4$^+$ cells
derived from transduced CD34$^+$ precursor cells were challenged with
SIVmac$_{239}$, an SIV strain that replicates well in T cells, at an MOI of
10^{-2}. Twenty-one days post infection, there was no detectable SIV
replication (<50 pg of SIV p27/ml) in the CD4$^+$ T cells containing
the *antitat* gene. Control CD4$^+$ cells containing only the *npt* gene
showed SIV p27 levels exceeding 20 ng/ml. At 21 days post-infection,
the CD4$^+$ *antitat* containing cells remained viable, while control cells
showed marked cytopathic effects (27% viability +/- 17%). Macrophage-like cells derived from CD34$^+$ cells transduced with *antitat*
were challenged with the macrophage tropic SIVmac$_{316}$, at an MOI
of 10^{-3}. These cells showed no detectable SIV replication, while control cells showed SIV p27 antigen levels of greater than 20 ng/ml at
12 days. Human CD4$^+$ T cells derived from CD34$^+$ cells transduced
with *antitat* were challenged with a stock of HIV-1 derived from the
NL4-3 molecular clone. At 14 days postinfection, there was no detectable viral replication, while control cells showed HIV-1 p24 levels of greater than 10 ng/ml. Despite the apparent success of the
antitat gene in inhibiting SIV and HIV-1 replication, it must be noted
that viral replication in control cells was very modest. Nevertheless,
this work provides the basis for developing primate animal models
of AIDS gene therapy in the future.

Strengths and Weaknesses of Primate Models
The close genetic relationship between monkeys and humans
makes the monkey an appropriate model in which to test preclinical
therapies for AIDS. Although transduction of human hemopoietic
stem cells with mouse retroviral vectors, with subsequent differentiation of these transduced cells, has achieved a higher rate of success in SCID-hu mice than in primate models, retroviral vector-mediated gene transfer into primate HSC has been shown to be effective,
with expression of the retroviral gene products for up to three years
post BMT. In addition, post-BMT assessment of repopulation of the
primate grafts with transduced cells has yielded information on the
logistics of ex vivo transduction of autologous grafts as well as providing data on the potential risks of implanting replication compe-

tent retroviruses. Infection of CD4$^+$ cells derived from transduced CD34+ cells with SIVmac$_{239}$ in vitro should lead the way for future studies of therapeutic gene transfer into primate HSC with in vivo differentiation of CD34$^+$ cells. The use of SIV rather than HIV-1 will remain a limitation of this system, since potential gene therapeutic agents may not be directly transferable from one system to the other.

Summary

Considerable progress has been made in developing animal models to test gene therapeutic agents targeted at HIV-1. In particular, SCID-mice bearing human hemopoietic cells transduced with marker genes and AIDS gene therapeutic agents are now being used in a number of laboratories. The value of these model systems lies in developing the technologies to efficiently transduce human hemopoietic stem cells and in the validity of these models for the study of HIV-1 pathogenesis. Much work remains to be done in both areas, but the transduction of human hemopoietic stem cells and their development into mature transduced T cells has been done more efficiently in SCID-hu mice than in any other setting. The reports by Goldstein of increased peripheral engraftment of human hemopoietic cells in SCID mice hold promise to make the SCID-hu mouse a more realistic model of HIV-1 pathogenesis and therefore also a better system to test AIDS gene therapies in the future. Primate models of gene therapy directed against SIV will surely be developed in the near future. While no good model of HIV-1 pathogenesis exists in a nonhuman primate species, SIV infection of macaques leads to a simian form of AIDS quite similar to human AIDS. This model system may also be fruitful in the development of techniques for transducing primate hemopoietic stem cells which will be applicable to the human system. Drawbacks of this system are that gene therapies directed against SIV may not be directly applicable to HIV-1 and that the many diverse HIV-1 isolates cannot be tested in this system. Nevertheless, the combination of primate and SCID-hu models should hasten the development and testing of gene therapy technologies and specific gene therapeutic agents for AIDS.

References

1. Berger EA. HIV entry and tropism: the chemokine receptor connection. AIDS 1997; 11:S3-S16.
2. Luciw P. Human immunodeficiency viruses and their replication. In: Fields BN, Knipe DM, Howley PM et al, eds. Fields Virology. 3rd ed. Philadelphia: Lippincott-Raven, 1996: 1881-1952.

3. Myers G, Korber B, Hahn BH et al. Human retroviruses and AIDS 1995. Los Alamos: Los Alamos National Laboratory, 1995.
4. Gardner MB, Luciw PA. Simian immunodeficiency viruses and their relationship to the human immunodeficiency viruses. AIDS 1988; 2 (suppl 1):S3-S10.
5. Bosma GC, Custer RP, Bosma MJ. A severe combined immunodeficiency mutation in the mouse. Nature 1983; 301:527-530.
6. Mosier DE, Gulizia RJ, Baird SM et al. Transfer of a functional human immune system to mice with severe combined immunodeficiency. Nature 1988; 335:256-259.
7. McCune JM, Namikawa R, Kaneshima H et al. The SCID-hu mouse murine model for the analysis of human hematolymphoid differentiation and function. Science 1988; 241:1632-1639.
8. Torbett BE, Picchio G, Mosier DE. hu-PBL-SCID mice: a model for human immune function, AIDS, and lymphomagenesis. Immunol Rev 1991; 124:139-164.
9. Carlsson R, Martensson C, Kalliomaki S et al. Human peripheral blood lymphocytes transplanted into SCID mice constitute an in vivo culture system exhibiting several parameters found in a normal humoral immune response and are a source of immunocytes for the production of human monoclonal antibodies. J Immunol 1992; 148:1065-107.
10. Mosier D, Gulizia R, Baird SM et al. Human immunodeficiency virus infection of human-PBL-SCID mice. Science 1991; 251:791-794.
11. Boyle MJ, Connors M, Flanigan ME et al. The human HIV/peripheral blood lymphocyte (PBL)-SCID mouse. J Immunol 1995; 154:6612-6623.
12. Mosier D, Gulizia RJ, MacIsaac P et al. Rapid loss of CD4+ T cells in human-PBL-SCID mice by noncytopathic HIV isolates. Science 1993; 260:689-692.
13. Connor R, Mohri H, Cao Y et al. Increased viral burden and cytopathogenicity correlate temporally with CD4+ T lymphocyte decline and clinical progression in HIV-1 infected individuals. J Virol 1993; 67:1772-1777.
14. Mosier DE, Gulizia RJ, MacIssac PD et al. Resistance to human immunodeficiency virus 1 infection of SCID mice reconstituted with peripheral blood lymphocytes from donors vaccinated with vaccinia gp 160 and recombinant gp 160. Proc Natl Acad Sci USA 1993; 86:2365-2369.
15. Woffendin C, Ranga, U, Yang Z et al. Expression of a protective gene prolongs survival of T cells in human immunodeficiency virus-infected patients. Proc Natl Acad Sci USA 1996; 93:2889-2894.
16. McCune JM. Development and applications of the SCID-hu mouse model. Seminars in Immunology 1996; 8:187-196.
17. Namikawa R, Weilbaecher KN, Kaneshima H et al. Long-term human hematopoiesis in the SCID-hu mouse. J Exp Med 1990; 172:1055-1063.

18. Stanley SK, McCune JM, Kaneshima H et al. HIV infection of the human thymus and disruption of the thymic microenvironment in the SCID-hu mouse. J Exp Med 1993; 178:1151-1163.

19. Aldrovandi GM, Feuer G, Gao L et al. The SCID-hu mouse as a model for HIV-1 infection. Nature 1993; 363 (6431):732-736.

20. Bonyhadi ML, Rabin L, Salimi S et al. HIV induces thymus depletion in vivo. Nature 1993; 363:728-736.

21. Jamieson BD, Aldrovandi GM, Planelles V et al. Requirement of HIV-1 *nef* for in vivo replication and pathogenicity. J Virol 1994; 68:3478-3485.

22. Deacon NJ, Tsykin A, Soloman A et al. Genomic structure of an attenuated quasi species of HIV-1 from a blood transfusion donor and recipients. Science 1995; 270:988-991.

23. Kaneshima H, Su L, Bonyhadi ML et al. Rapid-high, syncytium-inducing isolates of HIV-1 cytopathicity in the human thymus of the SCID-hu mouse. J Virol 1994; 68:8188-8192.

24. Akkina RK, Rosenblatt JD, Campbell AG et al. Modeling human lymphoid precursor cell gene therapy in the SCID-hu mouse. Blood 1994; 84:1393-1398.

25. Sutherland HJ, Lansdorp PM, Henkelman DH et al. Functional characterization of individual human hematopoietic stem cells cultured at limiting dilution on supportive marrow stromal layers. Proc Natl Acad Sci USA 1990; 87:3584-3588.

26. Champseix C, Maréchal V, Khazaal I et al. A cell surface marker gene transferred with a retroviral vector into CD34+ cord blood cells is expressed by their T cell progeny in the SCID-hu thymus. Blood 1996; 88(1):107-113.

27. An DS, Koyanagi Y, Zhao J-Q et al. High-efficiency transduction of human lymphoid progenitor cells and expression in differentiated T cells. J Virol 1997; 71(2):1397-1404.

28. Bonyhadi ML, Moss K, Voytovich A et al. RevM10-expressing T cells derived in vivo from transduced human hematopoietic stem-progenitor cells inhibit human immunodeficiency virus replication. J Virol 1997; 71(6):4707-4716.

29. Bevec D, Dobrovnik M, Hauber J et al. Inhibition of human immunodefiency virus type 1 replication in human T cells by retroviral-mediated gene transfer of a dominant-negative *rev* trans-activator. Proc Natl Acad Sci USA 1992; 89:9870-9874.

30. Malim MH, Freimuth WW, Liu J et al. Stable expression of transdominant Rev protein in human T cells inhibits human immunodefiency virus replication. J Exp Med 1992; 176:1197-1201.

31. Kyoizumi S, Baum C, Kaneshima H et al. Implantation and maintenance of functional human bone marrow into SCID-hu mice. Blood 1992; 79:1704-1711.

32. Chen BP, Galy A, Kyoizumi S et al. Engraftment of human hematopoietic precursor cells with secondary transfer potential in SCID-hu mice. Blood 1994; 84(8):2497-2505.

33. Su L, Lee R, Bonyhadi M et al. Hematopoietic stem cell-based gene therapy for acquired immunodeficiency syndrome: efficient transduction and expression of RevM10 in myeloid cells in vivo and in vitro. Blood 1997; 89(7):2283-2290.

34. Kamel-Reid S, Dick JE. Engraftment of immune deficient mice with human hematopoietic stem cells. Science 1988; 242:1706-1709.

35. Lapidot T, Pflumio F, Doedens F et al. Cytokine stimulation of multilineage human hematopoiesis from immature cells transplanted into SCID mice. Science 1992; 255:1137-1141.

36. Kollmann TR, Kim A, Zhuang X et al. Multilineage hematopoiesis and peripheral reconstitution of SCID mice with human lymphoid and myeloid cells following transplantation with human fetal bone marrow. Proc Natl Acad Sci USA 1994; 91:8032-8036.

37. Yurasov S, Kollmann TR, Kim A et al. SCID mice engrafted with human T cells, B cells, and myeloid cells after transplantation with human fetal bone marrow or liver cells and implanted with human fetal thymus: a model for studying human gene therapy. Blood 1997; 89 (5):1800-1810.

38. Laurent-Crawford AG, Drust B, Muller S et al. The cytopathic effect of HIV is associated with apoptosis. Virology 1991; 185:829-839.

39. Terai C, Kornbluth RS, Pauza CD et al. Apoptosis as a mechanism of cell death in cultured lymphoblasts acutely infected with HIV-1. J Clin Invest 1991; 87:1710-1715.

40. Walker BD, Chakrabarti S, Moss B et al. HIV-specific cytotoxic T lymphocytes in seropositive individuals. Nature 1987; 328:345-348.

41. Tanneau R, McChesney M, Lopez O et al. Primary cytotoxicity against the envelope glycoprotein of human immunodeficiency virus-1: evidence for antibody-dependent cellular cytotoxicity in vivo. J Infec Dis 1990; 162:837-843.

42. Gary RF. Potential mechanisms for the cytopathic properties of HIV. AIDS 1989; 3:683-694.

43. Lifson JD, Feinberg MB, Reyes GR et al. Induction of CD4-dependent cell fusion by the HTLV-III/LAV envelope glycoprotein. Nature 1986; 323:725-728.

44. Su L, Kaneshima H, Bonyhadi M. HIV-1 induced thymocyte depletion is associated with indirect cytopathicity and infection of progenitor cells in vivo. Immunity 1995; 2:25-36.

45. Jamieson BD, Uittenbogaart CH, Schmid I et al. High viral burden and rapid CD4+ cell depletion in human immunodeficiency virus type 1-infected SCID-hu mice suggest direct viral killing of thymocytes in vivo. J Virol 1997; 71(11):8245-8253.

46. Fultz P, McClure H, Swenson R et al. Persistent infection of chimpanzees with human T-lymphotropic virus type III/lymphadenopathy-associated virus: a potential model for acquired immunodeficiency syndrome. J Virol 1986; 58; 116-124.

47. Fultz P, McClure H, Swenson R et al. HIV infection of chimpanzees as a model for testing chemotherapeutics. Intervirology 1989; 30S1:51-58.

48. Agy MB, Frumkin LR, Corey L et al. Infection of *Macaca nemestrina* by human immunodeficiency virus type-1. Science 1992; 257:103-106.

49. Letvin NL, Daniel MD, Sehgal PK et al. Induction of AIDS-like disease in macaque monkeys with T cell tropic retrovirus STLV-III. Science 1985; 230:71-73.

50. van Beusechem VW, Valerio D. Gene transfer into hematopoietic stem cells of nonhuman primates. Human Gene Therapy 1996; 7:1649-1668.

51. van Bekkum DW. The rhesus monkey as a preclinical model for bone marrow transplantation. Transplant Proc 1978; 10:105-111.

52. Anderson WF, Kantoff P, Eglitis M et al. Gene transfer and expression in nonhuman primates using retroviral vectors. In: Cold Spring Harbor Symp Quant Biol 1986; 51:1073-1081.

53. Kantoff PW, Gillio AP, McLachlin JR et al. Expression of human adenosine deaminase in nonhuman primates after retrovirus-mediated gene transfer. J Exp Med1987; 166:219-234.

54. Cornetta K, Wieder R, Anderson WF. Gene transfer into primates and prospects for gene therapy in humans. Prog Nucl Acid Res Mol Biol 1990; 36:311-322.

55. Bodine DM, McDonagh KT, Brandt SJ et al. Development of a high-titer retrovirus producer cell line capable of gene transfer into rhesus monkey hematopoietic stem cells. Proc Natl Acad Sci USA 1990; 87:3738-3742.

56. van Beusechem VW, Kukler A, Einerhand M et al. Expression of human ADA in mice transpalnted with hemopoietic stem cells infected with amphotropic retroviruses. J Exp Med 1990; 172:729-736.

57. Andrews RG, Bryant EM, Bartelmez SH et al. CD34+ marrow cells, devoid of T and B lymphocytes, reconstitute stable lymphopoiesis and myelopoiesis in lethally irradiated allogenic baboons. Blood 1992; 80:1693-1701.

58. Xu LC, Karlsson S, Byrne ER et al. Long-term in vivo expression of the human glucocerebrosidase gene in nonhuman primates after CD34+ hematopoietic cell transduction with cell-free retroviral vector preparations. Proc Natl Acad Sci USA 1995; 92:4372-4376.

59. Kaptein LCM, van Beusechem VW, Riviere I et al. Long-term in vivo expression of the MFG-ADA retroviral vector in rhesus monkeys transplanted with transduced bone marrow cells. Hum Gene Ther 1997; 8:1605-1610.

60. van Beusechem VW, Kukler A, Heidt PJ et al. Long-term expression of human adenosine deaminase in rhesus monkeys transplanted with retrovirus-infected bone-marrow cells. Proc Natl Acad Sci USA 1992; 89:7640-7644.

61. Gerritsen WR, Wagemaker G, Jonker M et al. The repopulation capacity of bone marrow grafts following pretreatment with monoclonal antibodies against T lymphocytes in rhesus monkeys. Transplantation 1988; 45:301-307.

62. Kingston R, Jenkinson EJ, Owen JJT. A single stem cell can recolonize an embryonic thymus producing phenotypically distinct T cell populations. Nature 1985; 317:811-813.

63. van Ewijk W. T cell differentiation is influenced by thymic microenvironments. Annu Rev Immunol 1991; 9:591-615.

64. Rosenzweig M, Marks DF, Zhu H et al. In vitro T lymphopoiesis of human and rhesus CD34+ progenitor cells. Blood 1996; 87: 4040-4048.

65. Haynes BF, Denning S, Le PT et al. Human intrathymic T cell differentiation. Semin Immunol 1990; 2:67-77.

66. Terstappen WMM, Huang S, Picker LJ. Flow cytometric assessment of human T cell differentiation in thymus and bone marrow. Blood 1990; 70:666-677.

67. Haynes BF, Martin ME, Kay HH. Early events in human T cell ontogeny. J Exp Med 1988; 168:1061-1080.

68. Reimann KA, Waite BCD, Lee-Parritz DE et al. Use of human leukocyte-specific monoclonal antibodies for clinically immunophenotyping lymphocytes of rhesus monkeys. Cytometry 1994; 17:102-108.

69. Rosenzweig M, Marks DF, Hempel D et al. In vitro lymphopoiesis: a model system for stem cell gene therapy in AIDS. J Med Primatol 1996; 25:192-200.

70. Rosenzweig M, Marks DF, Hempel D et al. Transduction of CD34+ hematopoietic progenitor cells with an *antitat* gene protects T cell and macrophage progeny from AIDS infection. J Virol 1997; 71: 2740-2746.

CHAPTER 8

Hematopoietic Stem Cell Transplantation and HIV Gene Therapy

Clay Smith and Cristina Gasparetto

Introduction

Successful transplantation of gene modified hematopoietic stem cells is central to achieving durable replacement of the hematopoietic and immune systems with gene modified cells resistant to HIV infection. Enormous strides have been made in understanding the biology of hematopoietic stem cell transplantation over the last twenty years, in identifying a variety of hematopoietic stem cells and in minimizing the toxicity and expense of hematopoietic stem cell transplantation. In this review, we will summarize the biology of hematopoietic stem cell transplantation as well as highlight some of the clinical considerations that are relevant to stem cell based approaches to HIV gene therapy.

Principles of Hematopoietic Stem Cell Transplantation

It is now clear that hematopoiesis is maintained by a small population of cells termed pluripotent hematopoietic stem cells (PHSCs).[1,2] These cells can generate all hematopoietic lineages and have a very high self renewal potential. PHSCs generate a variety of progeny with progressively limited potential to self renew and generate different cell lineages. At least in mice, a single PHSC can reconstitute the entire hematopoietic system for the lifetime of the animal.[3] In contrast, more committed stem cells generate progeny for only limited periods of time.[4,5] Consequently, PHSCs must be present in the

Gene Therapy for HIV Infection, edited by Clay Smith. © 1998 Springer-Verlag and R.G. Landes Company.

transplant innoculum to durably reconstitute the recipient. For HIV gene therapy approaches, it is critical that the PHSCs be efficiently transduced with vectors encoding the HIV inhibitor. It may be useful to include more committed stem cells in the transplant innoculum, since these cells may generate terminally differentiated cells, particularly neutrophils and platelets, more quickly than PHSCs. Since neutrophils are critical to the management of bacterial infections, and platelets are critical in controlling bleeding, the contribution of committed cells to more rapid engraftment could be critical in reducing the complications of transplantation. In addition, there is some evidence that a subset of lymphoid cells termed "facilitator cells" may enhance PHSC engraftment, at least in some settings.[6] Hematopoietic stem cells have been identified in a variety of tissues, including bone marrow, peripheral blood and umbilical cord blood.[7-11] Autologous and allogeneic stem cells from each of the sources have been used to transplant and reconstitute the hematopoietic and immune systems. In addition, fetal liver stem cells have been used to transplant a small number of recipients.[12,13]

Autologous Bone Marrow and Peripheral Blood Stem Cell Transplantation

Autologous stem cell transplantation has been pioneered over the last decade in patients with malignancies using high doses of chemotherapy and/or radiotherapy.[14-16] In many patients at high risk for disease relapse, administration of high doses of chemotherapy and/or radiotherapy (termed the conditioning regimen) followed by autologous hematopoietic stem cell transplantation appears to be more effective than administration of standard dose chemotherapy at inducing tumor remissions and preventing relapse. Common chemotherapeutic agents used in the conditioning regimens for autologous transplants include cyclophosphamide, thiotepa, carmustine (BCNU), cis-platinum, and etoposide, among others. One of the primary effects of these agents at high doses is long term or permanent marrow aplasia. Consequently, the patient must be rescued from this toxicity by transplanting autologous or allogeneic hematopoietic stem cells to re-establish the hematopoietic and immune systems. In order to accomplish this, hematopoietic cells are collected prior to treatment with the conditioning regimen, cryopreserved and then re-infused into the patient after myeloablation. Autologous transplantation has been widely used in the treatment of hematologic diseases including lymphoma, multiple myeloma, as well as in some solid tumors including breast cancer and brain tumors.[14-17]

Sources of Autologous Hematopoietic Stem Cells

Initially, autologous bone marrow was used as the source of hematopoietic stem cells to re-establish the hematopoietic system following myeloablative radiotherapy and/or chemotherapy. In the past several years, stem cells circulating in the peripheral blood (peripheral blood stem cells or PBSCs) have been increasingly utilized for autologous transplantation.[18,19] PBSCs are typically collected by leukapheresis following treatment with chemotherapy and/or the administration of cytokines such as G-CSF and GM-CSF.[20-22] Chemotherapy and cytokines serve to mobilize bone marrow stem cells into the peripheral blood. These mobilized PBSCs are substantially enriched for hematopoietic stem cells compared to baseline circulating PBSCs. The advantages to using mobilized autologous PBSCs relative to bone marrow or nonmobilized PBSCs to re-establish hematopoiesis following high dose therapy include more rapid engraftment, decreased transfusion requirements, and diminished transplant related toxicity.[20-22] Neutrophils typically engraft in approximately 8-14 days and platelets typically engraft in 12-20 days following autologous PBSC transplantation, although there can be substantial individual variation.[19,23] Based on these advantages, some institutions have recently been able to perform autologous PBSC transplants in the outpatient setting.[21] This has substantially improved quality of life for patients and reduced the expense of the procedure. While initially there were concerns that transplantation of PBSCs would not durably sustain hematopoiesis following transplantation, studies conducted over the last few years involving transplantation of allogeneic peripheral blood stem cells indicates that PBSCs are capable of durably sustaining hematopoiesis for at least several years, if not permanently.[24-26] In addition, several studies have now shown that autologous PBSCs which have been enriched for primitive hematopoietic stem cells through immunoabsorption or flow cytometry can rapidly and consistently engraft patients with a variety of malignancies.[27-30]

Toxicities Associated with Autologous Stem Cell Transplantation

There are a number of toxicities associated with autologous transplantation which contribute to the morbidity and mortality of this procedure. Most of these are related to the high doses of radiotherapy and/or chemotherapy and are not due to the autologous stem cell transplant per se. The primary toxicities of autologous stem cell transplantation include infections due to neutropenia, bleeding, hepatic veno-occlusive disease, renal insufficiency or failure, pulmonitis or pulmonary hemorrhage, and mucositis. Virtually all patients have nausea, vomiting and anorexia.

Infections occur primarily as a consequence of the neutropenia which occurs after administration of the conditioning regimen.[31,32] Common infections following transplantation include gram negative and gram positive bacterial sepsis, primarily derived from damaged gastrointestinal tissue and from the large bore intravenous catheters placed for administering fluids, antibiotic, transfusions, and the stem cell infusion.[33-37] A variety of other bacterial infections including urinary tract infections, sinusitis, pneumonia, cellulitis, otitis, and dental abscesses can also occur.[38,39] *Candida* and other fungal species also cause a variety of infections including pneumonia, sepsis, sinusitis and hepatosplenic infections.[40,41] Viral infections including mucocutaneous herpes simplex virus infections as well as pneumonia, hepatitis, and bone marrow suppression from cytomegalovirus (CMV) also occur.[42-44] Rarely, parasitic infections including *Pneumocystis carinii* pneumonia and *Strongyloides* hyperinfection are seen after autologous transplantation.[45-47] Frequently, the clinical signs and symptoms of these infections are minimal during the period of neutropenia which occurs for one to three weeks following reinfusion of the stem cells, so a high degree of clinical suspicion must be maintained at all times. Prophylactic antibiotics are frequently administered during the period of pancytopenia, and intravenous antibiotics as well as anti-fungal and anti-viral agents are rapidly instituted when active infections are suspected.[40,44,48-50]

Bleeding occurs primarily from low platelet counts (thrombocytopenia) and/or coagulation factor deficiencies. Thrombocytopenia can be due to the conditioning regimen or to immune mediated platelet destruction. Platelet function can also be adversely affected by certain chemotherapies.[51] Clotting factor deficiencies may be due to liver damage, diffuse intravascular coagulation from infections or cancer, a reduction in vitamin K from poor nutrition or the effects of antibiotics on vitamin K producing bacteria in the GI tract, and occasionally from autoimmune processes directed at coagulation factors.[52] Bleeding can be catastrophic if it occurs in the lungs or intracerebrally. Other common sites of bleeding include the GI tract, nose, and urinary tracts. Bleeding is treated with platelet and red blood cell transfusions, administration of vitamin K, and occasionally, transfusion of coagulation factors.

Hepatic veno-occlusive disease (VOD) is caused by damage to endothelial cells, sinusoids, and hepatocytes of the liver from the conditioning regimen. The clinical signs of VOD include hepatomegaly, jaundice, and weight gain from fluid retention. The pathologic findings of VOD include fibrotic obliteration of venous lumens, hepatic congestion, hemorrhage, and hepatocyte disruption in a characteristic distribution. The severity of VOD ranges from mild to fatal. The diagnosis of VOD is typically made on clinical grounds, although Doppler ultrasound examination of the liver for blood flow abnormalities or trans-jugular liver biopsy can be helpful. A variety of attempts have been made to prevent or treat VOD, including shielding the liver from irradiation, administering prophylactic low doses of the anticoagulant heparin and administration of the thrombolytic agent tissue plasminogen activator to treat patients with severe VOD.[53] While some clinical studies suggest the utility of each of these approaches, it remains unproven whether any of these strategies can consistently prevent or treat VOD.[54] In addition to VOD, a variety of other processes can damage the liver after transplantation including drugs, viral infections, autoimmune processes and parenteral nutrition.

Renal insufficiency or failure occurs frequently after transplantation from the toxic effects of the conditioning regimen, antibiotics, other drugs, autoimmune processes and infections.[54,55] In addition, the kidneys can be damaged by a process termed thrombocytopenic thrombotic purpura (TTP) or a closely related process termed hemolytic uremic syndrome (HUS).[56-58] TTP or HUS typically does not occur until weeks or months after transplantation and can occur over a year after transplantation. In both TTP and HUS, fibrin deposition in the small arterioles and glomerular capillaries of the kidney lead to progressive renal insufficiency. In addition, platelet and red blood cell destruction occurs as blood circulates through the occluded renal blood vessels, leading to thrombocytopenia and anemia. In TTP, but not HUS, a similar process occurs in the brain, resulting in central nervous system dysfunction and fever. The etiology of TTP and HUS after transplantation is unknown; however direct damage to endothelial cells from the conditioning regimen which activates the clotting cascade and/or immune mediated processes may be responsible. TTP and HUS following transplantation can be treated with plasma exchange; however, this approach is frequently unsuccessful.[59] Paradoxically, the administration of platelets can worsen TTP or HUS, but platelet infusions may be unavoidable in patients with serious bleeding.

Pulmonary damage is common after transplantation and can occur through a variety of mechanisms. These include infections, pulmonary hemorrhage, pulmonary edema from volume overload or cardiac dysfunction, direct damage to the alveoli from irradiation and chemotherapy, veno-occlusive disease of the pulmonary circulation, and autoimmune mediated damage.[39,60,61] A distinct entity termed diffuse alveolar hemorrhage (DAH) can occur during the first few weeks after transplantation.[62] DAH is typically characterized by the abrupt onset of shortness of breath and decreased blood oxygen levels and is commonly associated with fungal infections. Diffuse pulmonary infiltrates are seen on chest X-ray exams. Bronchoalveolar lavage (BAL) is frequently necessary to distinguish DAH from other pulmonary processes with the same symptoms and signs. DAH may respond to treatment with steroids.[63] A delayed form of pneumonitis characterized by fever, weakness, shortness of breath, and pulmonary infiltrates is commonly seen several months after transplant in patients who received BCNU or irradiation as part of their conditioning regimen.[64] Reduction in the pulmonary diffusion capacity is characteristically seen on pulmonary function tests. Early treatment of this entity with steroids is frequently beneficial.

Other toxicities occurring after transplantation include cardiac damage resulting in heart failure or pericardial fluid collections, hypothyroidism or hypopituitarism, a variety of neurologic problems, sterility, alopecia, and secondary malignancies. Most of these toxicities are directly attributable to the conditioning agents.[65,66] Despite all of these potential toxicities, autologous transplantation is much less morbid than allogeneic transplantation, with an overall mortality of between 3 to 15% in recent series.

Allogeneic Bone Marrow and Peripheral Blood Stem Cell Transplantation

Autologous transplantation is not always feasible if the autologous stem cell collection contains large numbers of tumor cells which could be returned to the patient.[17] In addition, the patient's marrow may be hypoplastic from prior chemotherapy treatment, infections, or the underlying disease process, so that insufficient autologous stem cells can be collected to ensure engraftment. Allogeneic transplantation may also be preferable for some diseases such as chronic myelogenous leukemia (CML), where donor immune cells, including T lymphocytes and NK cells, appear to be capable of suppressing growth of the tumor. This has been termed a graft versus leukemia (GvL) or graft versus tumor (GvT) effect.[67,68] In developing stem cell based HIV gene therapy approaches, autologous transplantation may have several additional drawbacks. First, autologous marrow stem cells are frequently damaged during the course of HIV-1 disease by cytokines or HIV-1 proteins secreted by infected monocytes and T cells.[69-71] In addition, while the preponderance of evidence indicates that pluripotent stem cells are not infected directly with HIV-1, this issue has not been definitively settled.[70,72-74] Furthermore, even if HIV does not infect primitive hematopoietic cells, marrow and peripheral blood contains a large number of T cells and monocyte/macrophages that can house HIV.[75] Despite the development of immunoadherence based large scale methods for directly isolating CD34+ hematopoietic stem cells, and a variety of methods for depleting several log orders of T cells from marrow (see below), none of these methods are sufficiently effective to result in a transplant innoculum which is devoid of HIV infected cells. Consequently, it is likely that HIV-1 infected cells would be returned to the recipient following myeloablation. This would be irrelevant in patients who already have a substantial endogenous viral burden at the time of transplant. As described below, however, myeloablative therapy combined with effective combination antiretroviral therapy may substantially reduce the endogenous HIV burden so that returning large numbers of HIV infected cells could be a clinically important issue. One promising technology which may obviate this problem is the development of flow cytometric techniques for preparing highly purified populations of stem cells for gene therapy and transplantation purposes, devoid of HIV infected cells.[76] To use this technology, however, a transplant center would have to have a clinical grade flow sorter which can handle HIV infected samples, a limitation to the widespread use of this technology.

Toxicities Associated with Allogeneic Transplantation

Graft Rejection and Graft versus Host Disease (GvHD)

The incidence of toxicities and death is much higher in allogeneic transplantation than autologous transplantation. All of the toxicities described above for autologous transplantation occur after allogeneic transplantation, many with increased incidence and severity. Allogeneic transplantation is also associated with additional significant toxicities, including graft rejection and GvHD.[77-80] The incidence of graft rejection and graft versus host disease is primarily dependent on the HLA disparity between the donor and recipient.[80-84] In order to minimize the incidence and severity of GvHD and graft rejection, most allogeneic transplant donors and recipients are closely matched at the 3 pairs of HLA-A, B, and DR loci (i.e., a 6/6 HLA match). Minor histocompatability antigens, which can be virtually any cellular protein, may also contribute to graft rejection and GvHD. Consequently, the ideal allogeneic transplant donor is a syngeneic (identical) twin where all HLA and non-HLA antigens are identical to the recipient.[82] A 6/6 HLA matched sibling, which can be found for 10-25% of all patients, is the next most ideal donor. The incidence of graft rejection of 6/6 HLA matched or 5/6 HLA matched sibling transplants is <1% if the graft is not T cell depleted, and the incidence of severe acute GvHD is 20-40%.[83] Beyond this degree of HLA mismatch, the incidence of GvHD rises substantially, so that frequently either T cell depletion of the donor graft or identification of alternative donors is undertaken.[85] T cell depletion techniques and alternative donor sources of allogeneic hematopoietic stem cells are described in greater detail below.

Two forms of GvHD are seen after allogeneic transplantation, acute GvHD and chronic GvHD.[77-79] Acute GvHD is characterized by a maculopapular erythematous skin rash, fever, diarrhea, liver abnormalities, and marrow suppression and typically occurring 10-90 days after the transplant.[83] In addition to HLA disparity, another significant risk factor for the development of acute GvHD is age. Persons over 50 years of age have a risk of moderate to severe acute GvHD which can be as high as 80% in some studies, even in

HLA matched sibling transplants.[86,87] Acute GvHD is graded according to the amount of rash, diarrhea, and jaundice. Severe acute GvHD
can be treated with steroids, anti-thymocyte globulin, and antibodies directed at T cells.[83,88-90] Unfortunately, many cases of severe acute
GvHD do not respond to these treatments. Many patients with acute
GvHD develop chronic GvHD, although not all do. Chronic GvHD
typically occurs >100 days after transplantation and is characterized by skin changes ranging from superficial plaques to erythematous rashes to extensive fibrosis and sclerodermatous changes.[83]
These can lead to hair loss, decreased sweating, diminished mouth
and eye lubrication, and in some cases to joint contractures and severe disability. Other manifestations of chronic GvHD include liver
damage, weight loss, and obstructive pulmonary disease. Chronic
GvHD is treated with long termed steroid administration and/or ATG,
cyclosporine, and azathioprine.[89] A variety of other therapies, including low dose total lymphoid irradiation and thalidomide may
also benefit some patients with chronic GvHD.[90]

Methods for Minimizing Graft versus Host Disease

Since all patients receiving an allogeneic BMT from any donor
other than an identical twin are at substantial risk for severe GvHD,
a variety of methods have been developed as GvHD prophylaxis and
treatment. These include administration of the immunosuppressive
agents cyclosporine, methotrexate, or corticosteroids in the peri-
transplant period, or elimination of the T cells which mediate GvHD
from the transplant innoculum.[91-95] Administration of immunosuppressive agents causes a generalized immune suppression which results in a high incidence of opportunistic infections after transplantation (see below). In addition, steroids and cyclosporine have other
substantial toxicities, including significant effects on the central nervous system, bone density loss, renal impairment, and induction of
hypertension and hyperglycemia.

In order to avoid the complications of administering immunosuppressive agents, a variety of methods have been developed
for eliminating the T lymphocytes responsible for GvHD from the
allogeneic transplant innoculum.[68,91-93] Methods of T cell depletion
have included complement mediated lysis, immunotoxin treatment,
counterflow elutriation, monoclonal antibody immunoabsorbance,
and soybean agglutination combined with erythrocyte
rosetting.[94] The primary drawback to using T cell depletion for GvHD

prophylaxis is a higher rate of graft rejection and disease relapse compared to transplantation of whole bone marrow.[91] Graft failure occurring in T cell-depleted HLA mismatched BMT appears to be attributable mainly to immunologic rejection of donor hematopoietic cells by the host residual immune system.[95,96] Other mechanisms may play an important role as well, including competition between donor and residual host stem cells for the limited available niches in the bone marrow stroma and the homing efficiency of transplanted cells. In addition, immune reconstitution following T cell-depleted allogeneic transplantation may be not as robust as that seen following unmanipulated allogeneic transplantation.[97]

Opportunistic Infections After Allogeneic Transplantation

In addition to graft rejection and GvHD, allogeneic transplantation is associated with a higher incidence of opportunistic infections than autologous transplantation. The frequency and severity of these infections is higher than that following autologous transplantation for several reasons, including the administration of immunosuppressive agents to prevent or treat GvHD and the direct immunosuppressive actions of acute and chronic GvHD. In addition, while some aspects of immune function recover by 3-6 months, it typically takes over one year for most aspects of immune reconstitution to recover after allogeneic transplantation.[97-99] Immune reconstitution can be limited by both acute and chronic graft versus host disease.[100,101] Defects in immune reconstitution are typically more pronounced with increasing HLA disparity between the donor and recipient.

A particularly common infection following allogeneic transplantation is CMV pneumonitis.[102] This can be at prevented and treated in many cases by the administration of immunoglobulin and the anti-viral drug Gancyclovir.[103-105] Prophylactic immunoglobulin administration after allogeneic transplantation may also reduce the incidence and severity of other infections and acute GvHD as well.[106,107] The administration of Gancyclovir is frequently compromised by its myelosuppressive activities. CMV can also infect a variety of other organ systems, including the liver and bone marrow.[42] Other opportunistic infections seen after allogeneic transplantation include *P. carinii* pneumonia and reactivation of herpes zoster virus.[108] Chronically immunosuppressed allogeneic transplant recipients are also at greater risk for developing EBV related lymphoproliferative disorders.[109,110] Overall, the toxicities associated with allogeneic transplantation result in mortality rates of approximately 25% for this procedure.

Allogeneic Peripheral Blood Stem Cell Transplantation

As with autologous transplantation, allogeneic peripheral blood stem cells may be a useful alternative to bone marrow as the transplant source.[25,27,111-113] There are a number of potential advantages to using allogeneic PBSCs as opposed to allogeneic BM. First, tri-lineage engraftment may be more rapid with allogeneic PBSCs than when using bone marrow, diminishing the morbidity and expense associated with transplantation.[98,114-116] In particular, the incidence of infections occurring post transplant may be lessened. Second, a much higher dose of stem cells may be collected from the peripheral blood than from the bone marrow.[117] This may be critical for overcoming the high incidence of graft rejection observed in prior trials involving transplantation of T cell depleted bone marrow. Overcoming T cell depleted graft failure or rejection in HLA disparate donor/recipient pairs would also dramatically broaden the pool of available donors. The main theoretic disadvantage to using allogeneic PBSC is the potential for an increased risk of GvHD due to the presence of a log higher number of T cells in PBSC harvests relative to bone marrow.[118]

Alternative Allogeneic Donor Sources

In addition to obtaining allogeneic BM or PBSCs from HLA matched family members, allogeneic cells may be successfully transplanted from HLA matched but unrelated volunteer donors or from HLA haploidentical family donors.[27,92,119-123] HLA matched unrelated donor (MUD) bone marrow is obtained from volunteer donors who, through chance, have HLA similarity to the transplant recipient.[124] The ability to locate volunteer donors significantly broadens the availability of allogeneic transplants, since typically as few as 10-25% of all patients in the United States have a suitable HLA matched sibling donor. There are several problems associated with MUD transplants, however, including a several month lag in identifying and confirming a donor, and the high incidence of acute and chronic GvHD associated with this procedure.[125,126] This is probably due to significant minor histocompatability mismatches between the donor and recipient, as well as the fact that current HLA typing technologies do not typically determine if the HLA antigens of the donor and recipient are identical at every amino acid. Since even a single amino acid mismatch can lead to significant GvHD, complete genotype matching of bone marrow donors and recipients is desired but rarely found.[126]

Haploidentical family member donors, typically a mother or father, can be found for >90% of all potential transplant recipients.[117,121] Aversa et al recently reported treating 14 patients with end-stage chemo-resistant leukemia with transplantation of both bone marrow and G-CSF-mobilized peripheral blood progenitor cells from HLA haploidentical family members.[117] The average concentration of clonogenic stem cells in the final transplant innoculum was 7- to 10-fold greater than that found in bone marrow alone. The sole GvHD prophylaxis consisted of T cell depletion by the soybean agglutination and E-rosetting technique. The conditioning regimen included total body irradiation, ATG, cyclophosphamide and thiotepa. One patient rejected the graft, while the other 13 had early and sustained full-donor engraftment. These patients' neutrophils engrafted in a mean of 10 days, and platelets engrafted in a mean of 17 days. One patient, who received a much greater quantity of T lymphocytes than any other patient, died from grade IV acute GvHD. There were no other cases of GvHD among the evaluable patients. Four patients died from pneumonia (3 CMV, 1 idiopathic), 2 relapsed, and 6 patients are alive and well at a median follow-up of 4.5 months. These results indicate that haploidentical PBSC transplants may be a feasible and attractive alternative for patients who do not have an HLA matched sibling donor.

Umbilical Cord Blood Transplantation

Within the past decade, it was found that umbilical cord blood could serve as a source of hematopoietic stem cells for transplantation into both HLA matched sibling and unrelated recipients.[127-130] Umbilical cord blood (UCB) is obtained from placentas and typically cryopreserved prior to use, although some sibling transplants have used fresh UCB.[131-133] Several companies and institutions currently cryopreserve UCB for use in family members. Of much wider utility is the establishment of several volunteer donor UCB banks around the world.[132-136]

Fully or Partially HLA Matched Sibling Umbilical Cord Blood Transplantation

To date, umbilical cord blood from sibling and unrelated donors has been used to reconstitute hematopoiesis in more than 300 patients around the world with malignant and nonmalignant disorders. A summary of describing the outcome from 74 patients transplanted from full or partially HLA matched sibling UCB reported to the International Cord Blood Transplant Registry (ICBTR) has recently been presented.[137] For recipients of 6/6 or 5/6 HLA matched umbilical cord blood grafts, 91% of the patients engrafted. The median time to neutrophil recovery (defined as time to achieve an absolute neutrophil count (ANC) ≥ 5 x 10^8/L) and platelet recovery (define as platelet count ≥ 5 x 10^{10}/L untransfused for 7 days) was 22.0 days (range, 9 to 46) and 51 days (range, 15-117) after transplantation, respectively. Four patients never had signs of hematopoietic recovery and one patient had autologous recovery. Of the 5 patients without donor cell engraftment, 4 had undergone umbilical cord blood transplantation for the treatment of a bone marrow failure syndrome and one for the treatment of Hunter syndrome. Moderate to severe acute GvHD occurred in <5% of recipients of 6/6 or 5/6 HLA matched sibling umbilical cord blood transplants. Chronic GvHD was reported in only four patients and no patient had extensive disease. Of 15 recipients who had 4/6 and 3/6 partially HLA matched UCB transplants, 12 were evaluable for GvHD (3 died of graft failure). Moderate to severe GvHD occurred in 3. At a median follow-up of two years, 55% of the recipients of 6/6 or 5/6 HLA matched umbilical cord blood sibling UCB grafts were alive. Causes of death in the remainder included graft failure, malignancy relapse, interstitial pneumonitis/adult respiratory distress syndrome, veno-occlusive disease, intracranial hemorrhage, and bacterial sepsis. Only one patient died of GvHD.

Unrelated Fully or Partially HLA Matched UCB Transplantation in Children

Based on these encouraging experiences with fully or partially HLA matched sibling donor UCB transplantation, we and others have explored the use of unrelated UCB transplantation for both adults and children with hematologic malignancies, bone marrow failure states and congenital disorders.[129,138] Unrelated UCB is typically obtained from volunteer UCB banks established in New York, Milan,

Dusseldorf, Paris and London.[139] The National Heart Lung and Blood Institute of the NIH has recently expanded the UCB banking effort in the United States by funding new banks at Duke University Medical Center in Durham, North Carolina and elsewhere. Rubinstein et al summarized the results of the first 242 HLA matched or partially matched unrelated donor umbilical cord blood (MUD-UCB) transplants performed primarily in children between August 1993 and October 1996 facilitated by the new York Blood Center's Placental Blood Program.[140] Transplants were performed at 67 transplant centers worldwide (220 transplants in the U.S. and 52 transplants outside the U.S.). Transplants were performed as part of the treatment of malignant and nonmalignant disorders. Ninety percent of the evaluable patients engrafted. The median times to neutrophil and platelet recovery were 24 and 72 days, respectively. Of 163 patients surviving >100 days, severe acute GvHD occurred in 23%. Interestingly, the incidence of severe acute GvHD was not greater in recipients of 2 and 3 HLA antigen disparate grafts than in recipients of less disparate grafts. For recipients of a 6/6 or 5/6 HLA matched umbilical cord blood transplant, the probabilities of event-free survival at 3 years was approximately 50%.

Unrelated Umbilical Cord Blood Transplantation in Adults

Initially, because of the low total cell dose in UCB relative to BM and PBSCs, there was concern that related and unrelated UCB would fail to engraft in larger and older recipients. Several groups, including ours, have now demonstrated the feasibility of transplantation with related and unrelated UCB in larger children, adolescents, and adults.[141,142] We have recently reported our experience with 22 adult patients transplanted with unrelated UCB. The average weight of these patients was 69 kilograms (range 43-92 kg), and the average age was 32 years old (range 17-58 years). Virtually all patients had a high risk malignant or nonmalignant disorder and 7 of the patients had a prior bone marrow transplant. Only one patient was transplanted with HLA identical unrelated UCB, while sixteen received 4/6 partially HLA matched UCB. Patients received an average of 1.1×10^7 mononuclear cells/kg (range 0.6-3.7×10^7). Of the seventeen evaluable patients, the median time to neutrophil and platelet engraftment was 23 days (range 13-37 days) and 56 days (27-126 days) respectively. Severe GvHD occurred in three of the seventeen patients, while no to moderate GvHD occurred in the remainder. One patient developed chronic GvHD. Five patients died prior to evaluation for engraftment and GvHD from bacterial sepsis, multiorgan failure, and fungal infection. At a median follow-up of 211 days (range 43-909 days), 12 of the 22 patients were alive and free of disease. Ten of the patients had died, six from infections, two of GvHD, one from VOD, and one from a secondary lymphoproliferative disorder. These results suggest that unrelated HLA matched and partially matched UCB may engraft adults. In addition, as seen in children, the incidence and severity of GvHD appeared to be less than that seen with unrelated BM given the degree of HLA disparity.

In summary, UCB may have several significant advantages relative to MUD bone marrow as a source of stem cells for allogeneic transplant candidates lacking an appropriate sibling donor. These advantages include rapid availability of the UCB, ability to identify a donor for >85% of patients, absence of donor risk, and a very low risk of transmissible infectious diseases such as cytomegalovirus and Epstein-Barr virus. Other potential advantages include a lower risk of acute GvHD and the ability to expand the available donor pool in targeted ethnic and racial minorities currently underrepresented in all marrow donor registries. For HIV gene therapy purposes, there is also evidence that UCB stem cells are particularly amenable to ex vivo expansion and gene transfer.[143-148] Whether or not there truly is a reduced risk of GvHD for unrelated UCB transplantation relative to MUD-BM may have to be determined in randomized clinical trials, but the experience so far is promising. The biologic basis of the relatively reduced GvHD is unknown but may be due to processes which minimize fetal T cell reactivity against maternal tissue.

Clinical Experience with Stem Cell Transplantation in HIV Infected Persons

Given the toxicities of both autologous and allogeneic transplantation described above, it is clear that clinical trials of gene modified stem cells for the treatment of HIV infection must be undertaken judiciously. One clinical setting where the administration of myeloablative doses of chemotherapy and/or radiotherapy may be helpful in persons with HIV infection is in the treatment of relapsed or refractory AIDS related lymphoma.[149-151] Consequently, this clinical setting may offer an arena for exploring stem cell based gene therapy approaches to treating HIV infection as well. A small number of patients with AIDS related lymphoma (AIDS-NHL) have been treated in the past with allogeneic or syngeneic bone marrow transplantation.[152-161] Saral and Holland reported treating 8 patients with AIDS NHL with allogeneic (5 patients) or syngeneic (3 patients) BMT.[156,162] Seven patients received cyclophosphamide (CTX) (50 mg/kg x 4 d) and total body irradiation (TBI) (3 Gy/d x 4 d) and one patient received Busulfan (4 mg/kg x 4 d) and cyclophosphamide. All patients received intravenous zidovudine (AZT) for 2 weeks prior to BMT and oral AZT following BMT. All patients achieved at least a partial response (PR) with this treatment regimen. One patient died within 30 days of BMT. All the remaining patients survived greater than 30 days and achieved tri-lineage engraftment. Complete donor chimerism was noted in all allogeneic BMT recipients. Erythroid engraftment was slow in all patients and platelet recovery delayed in several. Two out of three allogeneic BMT recipients exhibited eradication of HIV by polymerase chain reaction (PCR) analysis following BMT (the remainder of the allo-BMT patients were not studied). One patient, who died at day +47 of recurrent lymphoma, was PCR negative for HIV in multiple tissues at autopsy. The second patient was HIV PCR negative from day +40 until day +120, when HIV recurred. This patient subsequently died of GvHD. These two patients received CTX/TBI and did not receive AZT prior to BMT. None of the three syngeneic BMT recipients demonstrated clearance of virus. Preliminary evidence indicated some correlation between the presence of AZT resistant virus at the time of BMT and failure to eradicate HIV. Immune reconstitution post BMT was not extensively evaluated in these patients. In another study, Aboulafia et al reported treating an HIV infected patient with a retroperitoneal B cell lymphoma with oral AZT, local radiation to the lymphoma and combinations of high dose chemotherapy prior to infusion of syngeneic bone marrow. Post-transplant, no GvHD was reported and engraftment occurred by day +18. A transient complete response was obtained; however, the patient died on day +52 of recurrent lymphoma.

In summary, the past clinical experience with allogeneic transplantation in patients with AIDS-related NHL indicates that persons with HIV infection can survive the myeloablative bone marrow transplant conditioning regimens and achieve reconstitution of the myeloid lineage. In addition, the intriguing finding was made that administration of irradiation and high doses of chemotherapy may have significantly reduced the HIV burden in some patients, at least transiently. This observation has been suggested in other studies as well.[163,164] Presumably, the reduced viral burden was due to elimination of HIV infected T cells or monocyte/macrophages by the myeloablative therapy. This raises the possibility that the transplant conditioning regimen used to ensure engraftment of donor cells may also contribute to the long term control of the viral burden. Further studies to determine the effects of myeloablative doses and even low doses of cytotoxic chemotherapy are clearly warranted to determine their effect on the HIV viral burden and reservoirs.

Potential Methods for Decreasing the Morbidity and Mortality of Stem Cell Transplantation in Persons with HIV Infection

If stem cell based approaches to HIV gene therapy which involve myeloablation are to be evaluated, techniques will need to be developed to minimize the toxicity associated with this procedure.

Prognostic Factors

One way for improving the outcome of stem cell transplantation in HIV infected persons would be to identify patients with prognostic factors indicating that they have a high chance of tolerating the transplant regimen. A review of the reported clinical trials involving treatment of patients with AIDS-NHL indicates that treatment outcome is correlated with several clinical prognostic features. Prognostic features which consistently appear to be useful for predicting which patients will tolerate a dose intensive form of therapy include a peripheral blood CD4 count of >200 cells/mm^3, a Karnofsky performance status >70%, and no history of AIDS defining illnesses.[165]

Improved Prophylaxis and Treatment of Post-Transplant Opportunistic Infections and HIV Infection

One approach to minimizing the transplant related toxicities is to vigorously prophylax and treat opportunistic infections arising in the post-transplant period. Significant advances have been made since the initial attempts to transplant allogeneic bone marrow into patients with HIV infection in this area. In particular, prophylaxis and treatment for CMV and *P. carinii* infections are increasingly being refined. In addition, significant advances have been made in the treatment of HIV infection which could reduce the chance for progressive HIV infection to occur in the post transplant period.

Numerous combinations of antiretroviral agents now appear to be able to suppress plasma HIV RNA levels below the lower limit of detection.[166] Most commonly, these combinations contain one or two nucleoside analog reverse transcriptase inhibitors with a protease inhibitor.[167,168] Other combinations which provide such potent suppression may also include two nucleoside reverse transcriptase inhibitors plus a nonnucleoside reverse transcriptase inhibitor or two protease inhibitors with or without nucleoside reverse transcriptase inhibitors. These effects can be achieved in both antiretroviral naive or experienced patient populations, although full suppression occurs most commonly and more durably in previously untreated persons. Consequently, it may be possible to administer multiple antiretroviral agents in the post transplant period to block HIV spread. Antiretroviral agents which are myelosuppressive, such as azidothymidine, may need to be avoided until engraftment has occurred, and intravenous preparations of antiretroviral agents may be necessary in the immediate post transplant period when patients have poor oral drug absorption due to mucositis or diarrhea.

Stem Cell Transplantation with Minimal Conditioning Regimens

To achieve consistent and high level engraftment of donor cells after transplantation, administration of doses of radiotherapy and/or chemotherapy is necessary.[169,170] As described above, administration of myeloablative doses of radiotherapy and/or chemotherapy is associated with substantial morbidity and mortality. Several strategies have been proposed to achieve partial engraftment of transplanted cells without using myeloablative conditioning regimens. In murine models, transplanting extremely high doses of whole bone marrow into untreated recipients can yield significant levels of engraftment for prolonged periods of time.[171-175] Currently, it remains unclear whether it is feasible to obtain sufficient cells from human donors to recapitulate this approach. In addition, it remains unclear whether this approach is restricted to only certain strains of mice as opposed to being a general phenomenon. In addition, gene therapy protocols will most likely use enriched stem cells rather than whole bone marrow to minimize the volume of vector needed to transduce the stem cells and to help improve the efficiency of gene transfer into these cells. While Nillson et al recently reported that highly purified stem cells could engraft untreated recipients, the level of engraftment was very low relative to engraftment achieved with whole bone marrow.[176] These studies indicated that engraftment of purified stem cells into untreated recipients may require the presence of nonstem cells which help facilitate engraftment.

Another strategy for achieving partial transplant chimerism is to treat the transplant recipient with nonmyeloablative doses of chemotherapy or radiotherapy. Mardiney et al demonstrated that significant levels of donor cell engraftment could be achieved in a murine model if the recipients were treated with sublethal doses of total body irradiation and transplanted with enriched stem cells. In addition, engraftment could be enhanced by pretreating recipient mice with G-CSF or G-CSF and stem cell factor.[177,178] The utility of this approach for stem cell based gene therapy applications was further demonstrated in a murine model of chronic granulomatous disease where biochemical and clinical improvements were observed after transplantation of gene modified stem cells. Champlin and his colleagues have used a sublethal chemotherapy-based conditioning regimen to achieve partial allogeneic engraftment, primarily with T cells, in patients with chronic lymphocytic leukemia.[179] Based on these observations, the use of sublethal conditioning may be a promising strategy for achieving partial but durable engraftment in recipients of gene modified autologous or allogeneic stem cells.

A third strategy for enhancing engraftment of gene modified stem cells without using myeloablative conditioning regimens is to include an in vivo selectable marker in the gene transfer vector. Examples of in vivo selectable markers include the multi-drug resistance (mdr) protein, which confers resistance to a number of chemotherapeutic agents including taxol, and mutant forms of the enzyme dihydrofolate reductase (DHFR), which confer resistance to drugs like methotrexate.[180-182] The goal of this strategy is to select for gene modified cells by administering taxol or methotrexate to recipients of gene modified cells in order to eliminate nontransduced cells. Ideally this would result in expansion in vivo of cells expressing the resistance gene. Proof of principle for this strategy has been demonstrated in murine models; however, this approach has not been confirmed so far in human studies.[183,184]

Prospects for Stem Cell Based Gene Therapy Approaches to Treating HIV Infection

Given the above discussion, what is the best way to develop and test stem cell based gene therapy approaches to treating HIV infection? At least several clinical scenarios can be proposed to test promising genetic HIV inhibitors via stem cell transplantation.

Transplantation of Autologous Gene Modified Peripheral Blood Stem Cells with a Sublethal Conditioning Regimen

This approach would be the most straightforward and least toxic approach to introducing gene modified stem cells into a person with HIV infection. The toxicities associated with a myeloablative regimen would be avoided, so that this approach could be tested in virtually any patient with HIV infection provided that they do not have damage to their endogenous hematopoietic stem cells. The primary disadvantage to this approach is that only a portion of the hematopoietic and immune system will be protected from HIV infection, since only partial donor engraftment can be expected even if all of the donor stem cells are genetically modified. If the extent of donor engraftment is low, then no clinical benefit could be expected to occur unless HIV infection itself would selectively eliminate nontransduced cells so that the gene modified cells progressively increased in proportion over time. If the genetic HIV inhibitor is effective, this approach could provide a reservoir of immunologically competent CD4+ T cells, as well as other hematopoietic cells which could provide some degree of immune competency. Combination antiretroviral agents would be continuously administered to control HIV replication as much as possible.

Transplantation of Autologous Gene Modified Umbilical Cord in Infants and Children with HIV Infection

In this strategy, UCB from an infant at risk for HIV infection from a seropositive mother is collected at delivery and either cryopreserved for later use or immediately transduced with an HIV resistance gene and transplanted. The gene modified UCB could be infused with a sublethal conditioning regimen as described above. Alternatively, if the infant or child demonstrated signs of rapidly progressive AIDS which was resistant to antiretroviral agents, a fully myeloablative regimen might be justified in an attempt to obtain full engraftment with gene modified cells.

Transplantation of Autologous or Allogeneic Gene Modified Peripheral Blood Stem Cells in Persons with Refractory or Relapsed AIDS Related Lymphoma

As described above, many HIV infected persons who develop AIDS related lymphoma may fail to respond to standard chemotherapy. Autologous or allogeneic transplantation may be a treatment option for patients who have prognostic factors suggesting that they may tolerate such an aggressive treatment approach. Autologous peripheral blood stem cell transplantation would be the least morbid approach but may be precluded if the patient's bone marrow is heavily involved with lymphoma or if insufficient stem cells can be collected. An alternative would be to perform allogeneic peripheral blood or bone marrow transplantation if the patient has an appropriate HLA matched sibling donor. If the patient does not have an appropriate sibling donor, fully or partially HLA matched unrelated donor umbilical cord blood transplantation could be an option. In either setting, the patient would be treated with as effective a combination of antiretroviral agents which could be identified following transplant in order to minimize infection of the transplanted cells. This clinical scenario could provide a setting for evaluating stem cell based HIV gene therapy with a fully myeloablative regimen. The advantage of this approach is that engraftment with gene modified donor cells would be higher than when sublethal conditioning regimens are used. The obvious disadvantage is the morbidity of using high dose radiation and/or chemotherapy. However, since the conditioning regimen would be used to treat the lymphoma, the patient would not be exposed to any further risk in order to engraft gene modified cells. An intriguing possible advantage to using myeloablation prior to transplanting gene modified cells is that it may contribute to reducing the reservoir of chronically infected long lived hematopoietic cells which appear to survive long term treatment with combinations of antiretroviral agents.[185] In the case where gene modified allogeneic cells from a healthy donor are transplanted, it may be possible to minimize the HIV burden in the patient even further. The combination of multiple antiretroviral agents, myeloablative therapy, allogeneic transplantation, and gene therapy could potentially be a potent multi-pronged approach to long term control of HIV infection.

In summary, stem cell based approaches to HIV gene therapy appear to be testable in a variety of clinical settings. Clearly however, the risks of any stem cell transplant procedure should be carefully considered. Consequently, premature clinical trials of stem cells transduced with genetic HIV inhibitors should not be undertaken unless they clearly demonstrate activity and safety in extensive preclinical testing. In addition, substantial limitations still exist in the ability to introduce novel genetic elements into the PHSCs which sustain hematopoiesis after transplantation.[146,186,187] Until these limitations are overcome, it is predictable that stem cell based approaches to HIV gene therapy will not be beneficial, because even if the genetic HIV inhibitor were fully effective, gene modified cells would not persist after transplantation. Despite these concerns, it remains only a matter of time before advances in vector design, ex vivo stem cell manipulation, and transplantation with novel sublethal conditioning regimens will make HIV gene therapy strategies testable in clinical trials. Ultimately, vectors may be designed which could deliver the genetic HIV inhibitors into hematopoietic stem cells or their progeny in vivo so that stem cell transplantation could be bypassed altogether.

References

1. Morrison SJ, Uchida N, Weissman IL. The biology of hematopoietic stem cells. [Review] [241 refs]. Annual Review of Cell & Developmental Biology 1995; 11:35-71.
2. Visser JW, de Vries P. Analysis and sorting of hematopoietic stem cells from mouse bone marrow. Methods in Cell Biology 1994; 42:243-61.
3. Osawa M, Hanada K, Hamada H, Nakauchi H. Long-term lymphohematopoietic reconstitution by a single CD34-low/negative hematopoietic stem cell. Science 1996; 273:242-5.
4. Morrison SJ, Weissman IL. Heterogeneity of hematopoietic stem cells: Implications for clinical applications. [Review] [30 refs]. Proceedings of the Association of American Physicians 1995; 107:187-94.
5. Weissman IL. Stem cells, clonal progenitors, and commitment to the three lymphocyte lineages: T, B, and NK cells [comment]. [Review] [17 refs]. Immunity 1994; 1:529-31.
6. Gaines BA, Colson YL, Kaufman CL, Ildstad S. Facilitating cells enable engraftment of purified fetal liver stem cells in allogeneic recipients. Experimental Hematology 1996; 24:902-13.
7. Almici C, Carlo-Stella C, Wagner JE, Rizzoli V. Umbilical cord blood as a source of hematopoietic stem cells: From research to clinical application. [Review]. Haematologica 1995; 80:473-9.

8. Amos TA, Gordon MY. Sources of human hematopoietic stem cells for transplantation—a review. [Review]. Cell Transplantation 1995; 4:547-69.

9. Henon P. Peripheral blood stem cell transplantations: past, present and future. Stem Cells 1993; 11:154-172.

10. Hong DS, Deeg HJ. Hemopoietic stem cells: sources and applications. [Review]. Medical Oncology 1994; 11:63-8.

11. Lu L, Shen RN, Broxmeyer HE. Stem cells from bone marrow, umbilical cord blood and peripheral blood for clinical application: Current status and future application. [Review]. Critical Reviews in Oncology-Hematology 1996; 22:61-78.

12. Touraine JL. Transplantation of fetal liver stem cells into patients and into human fetuses, with induction of immunologic tolerance. Transplantation Proceedings 1993; 25:1012-3.

13. Touraine JL. In utero transplantation of fetal liver stem cells into human fetuses. [Review] [15 refs]. Hematoth 1996; 5:195-9.

14. Philip T et al. High-dose therapy and autologous bone marrow transplantation after failure of conventional chemotherapy in adults with intermediate-grade or high-grade non-Hodgkin's lymphoma. The New England Journal of Medicine 1987; 316:1493-1498.

15. Hochberg FH, Parker LM, Takvorian T, Canellos GP, Zervas NT. High-dose BCNU with autologous bone marrow rescue for recurrent glioblastoma multiforme. Journal of Neurosurgery 1981; 54:455-60.

16. Nabholtz JM, al-Tweigeri T, Jacquelin N, Venner PM. Autologous bone marrow support and bone disease in metastatic breast cancer. [Review] [31 refs]. Canadian Journal of Oncology 1995; 5:369-75.

17. Lemoli RM, Cavo M, Fortuna A. Concomitant mobilization of plasma cells and hematopoietic progenitors into peripheral blood of patients with multiple myeloma. Journal of Hematotherapy 1996; 5:339-49.

18. Henon PR. Peripheral blood stem cell transplantation: Critical review. [Review] [40 refs]. International Journal of Artificial Organs 1993; 16:64-70.

19. To L et al.. Comparison of haematological recovery times and supportive care requirements of autologous recovery phase peripheral blood stem cell transplants, autologous bone marrow transplants and allogeneic bone marrow transplants. Bone Marrow Transplantation 1992; 9:277-284.

20. Murea S, Goldschmidt H, Hahn U, Pforsich M, Moos M, Haas R. Successful collection and transplantation of peripheral blood stem cells in cancer patients using large-volume leukaphereses. Journal of Clinical Apheresis 1996; 11:185-94.

21. Gilbert CJ. Peripheral blood progenitor cell transplantation for breast cancer: Pharmacoeconomic considerations. Pharmacotherapy 1996; 16:101S-108S.

22. Goldberg SL, Mangan KF, Klumpp TR, Macdonald JS, Thomas C, Mullaney MT, Au FC. Complications of peripheral blood stem cell harvesting: Review of 554 PBSC leukaphereses. [Review] [12 refs]. Journal of Hematotherapy 1995; 4:85-90.

23. Iacone A et al. Survival after PBSC transplantation and comparison of engraftment speed with autologous and allogeneic marrow transplantation: Results of a multicenter study. International Journal of Artificial Organs 1993; 5:45-50.

24. Janssen WE. Peripheral blood and bone marrow hematopoietic stem cells: are they the same? [Review]. Seminars in Oncology 1993.

25. Spitzer TR. Allogeneic peripheral blood stem cell transplantation. [Review]. Journal of Infusional Chemotherapy 1996; 6:33-8.

26. Bensinger WI, Appelbaum FA, Demirer T, Torok-Storb B, Storb R, Buckner CD. Transplantation of allogeneic peripheral blood stem cells. [Review] [56 refs]. Stem Cells 1995; 13:63-70.

27. Stockschlader M, Loliger C, Kruger W, Zeller W, Heyll A, Schonrock-Nabulsi P, Zander A. Transplantation of allogeneic rhG-CSF mobilized peripheral CD34+ cells from an HLA-identical unrelated donor. Bone Marrow Transplantation 1995; 16:719-22.

28. Chen BP et al. Cytokine-mobilized peripheral blood CD34+Thy-1+Lin- human hematopoietic stem cells as target cells for transplantation-based gene therapy. Leukemia 1995; 9:S17-25.

29. Korbling M et al. Large-scale preparation of highly purified, frozen/thawed CD34+, HLA-DR- hematopoietic progenitor cells by sequential immunoadsorption (CEPRATE SC) and fluorescence-activated cell sorting: implications for gene transduction and/or transplantation. Bone Marrow Transplantation 1994; 13:649-54.

30. Lebkowski JS, Schain L, Hall M, Wysocki M, Dadey B, Biddle W. Rapid isolation and serum-free expansion of human CD34+ cells. Blood Cells 1994; 20:404-10.

31. D'Antonio D, Iacone A, Pierelli L, Bonfini T. Patterns of recovery phase infection after autologous blood progenitor cell transplantation in patients with malignancies. The Gruppo Italiano di Studio per la Manipolazione Cellulare in Ematologia. European Journal of Clinical Microbiology & Infectious Diseases 1995; 14:552-6.

32. Emmanouilides C, Glaspy J. Opportunistic infections in oncologic patients. [Review] [83 refs]. Hematology—Oncology Clinics of North America 1996; 10:841-60.

33. LaRocco MT, Burgert SJ. Infection in the bone marrow transplant recipient and role of the microbiology laboratory in clinical transplantation. [Review] [312 refs]. Clinical Microbiology Reviews 1997; 10:277-97.

34. Sable CA, Donowitz GR. Infections in bone marrow transplant recipients. [Review] [7 refs]. Clinical Infectious Diseases 1994; 18:273-81; quiz 282-4.

35. Schimpff SC. Infection in bone marrow transplantation: a model for examining predisposing factors to infection in cancer patients. [Review] [27 refs]. Recent Results in Cancer Research 1993; 132:15-34.

36. Walter EA, Bowden RA. Infection in the bone marrow transplant recipient. [Review] [133 refs]. Infectious Disease Clinics of North America 1995; 9:823-47.

37. Crawford SW, Hickman RO, Ulz L, O'Quin T, Wong R, McDonald GB. Use of the Hickman-Crawford critical care catheter in marrow transplant recipients: A pulmonary artery catheter-adaptable central venous access [see comments]. Critical Care Medicine 1994; 22:347-52.

38. Yee S, Stern SJ, Hearnsberger HG, Suen JY. Sinusitis in bone marrow transplantation. Southern Medical Journal 1994; 87:522-4.

39. Winer-Muram HT, Gurney JW, Bozeman PM, Krance RA. Pulmonary complications after bone marrow transplantation. [Review] [36 refs]. Radiologic Clinics of North America 1996; 34:97-117.

40. Schuler U, Ehninger G. New approaches to the prophylaxis and treatment of bacterial and fungal infections in allogeneic marrow transplant recipients. [Review] [32 refs]. Bone Marrow Transplantation 1994; 14:S61-5.

41. Iwen PC, Kelly DM, Reed EC, Hinrichs SH. Invasive infection due to Candida krusei in immunocompromised patients not treated with fluconazole. Clinical Infectious Diseases 1995; 20:342-7.

42. Almeida-Porada GD, Ascensao JL. Cytomegalovirus as a cause of pancytopenia. [Review] [59 refs]. Leukemia & Lymphoma 1996; 21:217-23.

43. Galama JM, de Leeuw N, Wittebol S, Peters H, Melchers WJ. Prolonged enteroviral infection in a patient who developed pericarditis and heart failure after bone marrow transplantation. Clinical Infectious Diseases 1996; 22:1004-8.

44. Rayani SA, Nimmo CJ, Frighetto L, Martinusen SM, Nickoloff DM, Reece DE, Jewesson PJ. Implementation and evaluation of a standardized herpes simplex virus prophylaxis protocol on a leukemia/bone marrow transplant unit. Annals of Pharmacotherapy 1994; 28:852-6.

45. Dallorso S, Castagnola E, Garaventa A, Rossi GA, Giacchino R, Dini G. Early onset of Pneumocystis carinii pneumonia in a patient receiving bone marrow transplantation from a matched unrelated donor [letter]. Bone Marrow Transplantation 1994; 13:106-7.

46. Rotterdam H, Tsang P. Gastrointestinal disease in the immunocompromised patient. [Review] [214 refs]. Human Pathology 1994; 25:1123-40.

47. Castagnola E et al. Low CD4 lymphocyte count in a patient with P. carinii pneumonia after autologous bone marrow transplantation. Bone Marrow Transplantation 1995; 15:977-8.

48. Meisenberg B, Gollard R, Brehm T, McMillan R, Miller W. Prophylactic antibiotics eliminate bacteremia and allow safe outpatient management following high-dose chemotherapy and autologous stem cell rescue. Supportive Care in Cancer 1996; 4:364-9.

49. Momin F, Chandrasekar PH. Antimicrobial prophylaxis in bone marrow transplantation. [Review] [135 refs]. Annals of Internal Medicine 1995; 123:205-15.

50. Vossen JM, de Tollenaer S, van Weel-Sipman MH. Prophylaxis and pre-emptive therapy of bacterial infections following allogeneic bone marrow transplantation in children. Bone Marrow Transplantation 1996; 18:93-6.

51. Karolak L et a. High-dose chemotherapy-induced platelet defect: Inhibition of platelet signal transduction pathways. Molecular Pharmacology 1993; 43:37-44.

52. Seidler CW, Mills LE, Flowers ME, Sullivan KM. Spontaneous factor VIII inhibitor occurring in association with chronic graft-versus-host disease. [Review] [26 refs]. American Journal of Hematology 1994; 45:240-3.

53. Rio B, Bauduer F, Arrago JP, Zittoun R. N-terminal peptide of type III procollagen: A marker for the development of hepatic veno-occlusive disease after BMT and a basis for determining the timing of prophylactic heparin. Bone Marrow Transplantation 1993; 11:471-2.

54. Bearman SI, Lee JL, Baron AE, McDonald GB. Treatment of hepatic venocclusive disease with recombinant human tissue plasminogen activator and heparin in 42 marrow transplant patients. Blood 1997; 89:1501-6.

55. Haslam PJ, Proctor SJ, Goodship TH, Zouvani J. Immune complex glomerulonephritis, myasthenia gravis and compensated hypothyroidism in a patient following allogeneic bone marrow transplantation. Nephrology, Dialysis, Transplantation 1993; 8:1390-2.

56. Zeigler ZR et al. Plasma von Willebrand factor antigen (vWF:AG) and thrombomodulin (TM) levels in adult thrombotic thrombocytopenic purpura/hemolytic uremic syndromes (TTP/HUS) and bone marrow transplant-associated thrombotic microangiopathy (BMT-TM). American Journal of Hematology 1996; 53:213-20.

57. Wassmann B, Martin H, Elsner S, Bruecher J, Thaiss F, Stahl RA, Hoelzer D. Microangiopathic hemolytic anemia and renal impairment following autologous bone marrow transplantation: a case of hemolytic uremic syndrome? Bone Marrow Transplantation 1994; 14:849-51.

58. Ohno E, Ohtsuka E, Iwashita T, Uno N, Ogata M, Kikuchi H, Nasu M. Hemolytic uremic syndrome following autologous peripheral blood stem cell transplantation in a patient with malignant lymphoma. Bone Marrow Transplantation 1997; 19:1045-7.

59. Sarode R et al. Therapeutic plasma exchange does not appear to be effective in the management of thrombotic thrombocytopenic purpura/hemolytic uremic syndrome following bone marrow transplantation. Bone Marrow Transplantation 1995; 16:271-5.

60. Salzman D, Adkins DR, Craig F, Freytes C, LeMaistre CF. Malignancy-associated pulmonary veno-occlusive disease: report of a case following autologous bone marrow transplantation and review. [Review] [40 refs]. Bone Marrow Transplantation 1996; 18:755-60.

61. Garaventa A et al. Pneumopathy in children after bone marrow transplantation. Report from the AIEOP-BMT Registry. The Italian Association of Pediatric Hematology-Oncology BMT Group. Bone Marrow Transplantation 1996; 18:160-2.

62. Corso S, Vukelja SJ, Wiener D, Baker WJ. Diffuse alveolar hemorrhage following autologous bone marrow infusion. Bone Marrow Transplantation 1993; 12:301-3.
63. Metcalf JP, Rennard SI, Reed EC, Haire WD, Sisson JH, Walter T, Robbins RA. Corticosteroids as adjunctive therapy for diffuse alveolar hemorrhage associated with bone marrow transplantation. University of Nebraska Medical Center Bone Marrow Transplant Group. American Journal of Medicine 1994; 96:327-34.
64. Kantrow SP, Hackman RC, Boeckh M, Myerson D, Crawford SW. Idiopathic pneumonia syndrome: Changing spectrum of lung injury after marrow transplantation. Transplantation 1997; 63:1079-86.
65. Toubert ME et al. Short- and long-term follow-up of thyroid dysfunction after allogeneic bone marrow transplantation without the use of preparative total body irradiation. British Journal of Haematology 1997; 98:453-7.
66. Kubota C et al. Changes in hypothalamic-pituitary function following bone marrow transplantation in children. Acta Paediatrica Japonica 1994; 36:37-43.
67. Miyamura K, Barrett AJ, Kodera Y, Saito H. Minimal residual disease after bone marrow transplantation for chronic myelogenous leukemia and implications for graft-versus-leukemia effect: a review of recent results. [Review] [64 refs]. Bone Marrow Transplantation 1994; 14:201-9.
68. Okunewick JP, Kociban DL, Machen LL, Buffo MJ. Comparison of the effects of CD3 and CD5 donor T cell depletion on graft-versus-leukemia in a murine model for MHC-matched unrelated-donor transplantation. Bone Marrow Transplantation 1994; 13:11-7.
69. Calenda V, Chermann JC. The effects of HIV on hematopoiesis. Eur J Haematol 1992; 48:181-6.
70. Re M, Furlini G, Zauli G, La Placa M. Human immunodeficiency virus type 1 (HIV-1) and human hematopoietic progenitor cells. Archives of Virology 1994; 137:1-23.
71. Scadden DT. Hematologic disorders and growth factor support in HIV infection. [Review] [100 refs]. Hematology—Oncology Clinics of North America 1996; 10:1149-61.
72. Molina J, Scadden D, Sakaguchi M, Fuller B, Woon A, Groopman J. Lack of evidence for infection of or effect on growth of hematopoietic progenitor cells after in vivo or in vitro exposure to human immunodeficiency virus. Blood 1990; 76:2476-2482.
73. Kaushal S et al. Exposure of human CD34+ cells to human immunodeficiency virus type 1 does not influence their expansion and proliferation of hematopoietic progenitors in vitro. Blood 1996; 88:130-7.
74. Marandin A, Katz A, Oksenhendler E, Tulliez M, Picard F, Vainchenker W, Louache F. Loss of primitive hematopoietic progenitors in patients with human immunodeficiency virus infection. Blood 1996; 88:4568-78.

75. Poli G, Fauci A. The role of monocyte/macrophages and cytokines in the pathogenesis of HIV infection. Pathobiology 1992; 60:246-251.
76. Junker U et al. Hematopoietic potential and retroviral transduction of CD34+ Thy-1+ peripheral blood stem cells from asymptomatic human immunodeficiency virus type-1-infected individuals mobilized with granulocyte colony-stimulating factor. Blood 1997; 89:4299-306.
77. Bron D. Graft-versus-host disease. [Review] [51 refs]. Current Opinion in Oncology 1994; 6:358-64.
78. Chao NJ. Graft-versus-host disease: the viewpoint from the donor T cell. [Review] [82 refs]. Biology of Blood and Marrow Transplantation 1997; 3:1-10.
79. Ferrara JL, Cooke KR, Pan L, Krenger W. The immunopathophysiology of acute graft-versus-host-disease. [Review] [139 refs]. Stem Cells 1996; 14:473-89.
80. Kelemen E, Szebeni J, Petranyi GG. Graft-versus-host disease in bone marrow transplantation: Experimental, laboratory, and clinical contributions of the last few years. [Review] [151 refs]. International Archives of Allergy & Immunology 1993; 102:309-20.
81. Crawford SW, Longton G, Storb R. Acute graft-versus-host disease and the risks for idiopathic pneumonia after marrow transplantation for severe aplastic anemia. [Review] [31 refs]. Bone Marrow Transplantation 1993; 12:225-31.
82. Okunewick JP, Kociban DL, Machen LL, Buffo MJ. Effect of donor and recipient gender disparities on fatal graft-vs.-host disease in a mouse model for major histocompatibility complex-matched unrelated-donor bone marrow transplantation [see comments]. Experimental Hematology 1993; 21:1570-6.
83. Sullivan K. Graft-versus-host disease. In Bone Marrow Transplantation. (eds. Forman, S., Blume, K., & Thomas, E.) 339-362 (Blackwell Scientific Publishers, Boston, 1994).
84. Beatty PG. The immunogenetics of bone marrow transplantation. [Review]. Transfusion Medicine Reviews 1994; 8:45-58.
85. Beatty P, Clift R, Mickelson E et al. Marrow transplantation from related donors other than HLA-identical siblings. NEJM 1985; 313:765-771.
86. Sullivan K, Kopecky K, Buckner C, Storb R. Intravenous IgG to prevent graft versus host disease after bone marrow transplantation. N Engl J Med 1990; 323:705-712.
87. Nash R, Pepe M, Storb R et al. Acute graft versus host disease: Analysis of risk factors after allogeneic marrow transplantation and prophylaxis with cyclosporine and methotrexate. Blood 192; 80:1838-1845.
88. Oblon DJ, Felker D, Coyle K, Myers L. High-dose methylprednisolone therapy for acute graft-versus-host disease associated with matched unrelated donor bone marrow transplantation. Bone Marrow Transplantation 1992; 10:355-7.
89. Vogelsang GB. Acute and chronic graft-versus-host disease. [Review] [18 refs]. Current Opinion in Oncology 1993; 5:276-81.

90. Parker PM et al. Thalidomide as salvage therapy for chronic graft-versus-host disease. Blood 1995; 86:3604-9.

91. Kernan N. T cell depletion for prevention of Graft-versus-Host disease. in *Bone Marrow Transplantation*. (eds. Forman S, Blume K Thomas E.) 124-135 (Blackwell Scientific Publishers, Boston, 1994).

92. Ash R et al. Successful allogeneic transplantation of T cell depleted bone marrow from closely HLA-matched unrelated donors. The New England Journal of Medicine 1990; 322:485-494.

93. Feugier P et al.. Comparison of T cell depletion strategies from bone marrow, umbilical cord and peripheral blood using five separation systems. Hematology & Cell Therapy 1997; 39:67-73.

94. Reisner Y, Kirkpatrick D, Dupont B et al. Transplantation of acute leukemia with HLA-A and B nonidentical parental marrow cells fractionated with soybean agglutinin and sheep red blood cells. Lancet 1981; 2:327-331.

95. Patterson J, Prentice H, Brenner M et al. graft rejection following HLA matched T cell depleted bone marrow transplantation. Br J Hematology 1986; 6:221-230.

96. Kernan N, Flomenberg N, Dupont B et al. Graft rejection in recipients of T cell depleted HLA nonidentical transplants for leukemia: identification of host derived anti-donor allocytototxic lymphocytes. Transplantation 1987; 43:482-487.

97. Daly J, Rozans M, Smith B et al. Retarded recovery of functional T cell frequencies in T cell depleted bone marrow transplant recipients. Blood 1987; 70:960-964.

98. Roberts M, To L, Gillis D, Mundy J, Rawling C, Ng K, Juttner C. Immune reconstitution following peripheral blood stem cell transplantation, autologous bone marrow transplantation and allogeneic bone marrow transplantation. Bone Marrow Transplantation 1993; 12:469-475.

99. Duncombe AS et al. Bone marrow transplant recipients have defective MHC-unrestricted cytotoxic responses against cytomegalovirus in comparison with Epstein-Barr virus: The importance of target cell expression of lymphocyte function-associated antigen 1 (LFA1). Blood 1992; 79:3059-66.

100. Noel D, Witherspoon R, Storb R et al. Does GvHD influence the tempo of immunologic recovery after allogeneic bone marow transplantation? An analysis of long term survivors. Blood 1978; 51:1087-1105.

101. Seddik M, Seemayer T, Lapp W. The graft versus host reaction and immune function. Transplantation 1984; 37:281-286.

102. Meyers J, Flournoy N, Thomas E. Risk factors for cytomegalovirus infection after human marrow transplantation. J Inf Dis 1986; 153:478-488.

103. Goodrich JM, Boeckh M, Bowden R. Strategies for the prevention of cytomegalovirus disease after marrow transplantation. [Review] [93 refs]. Clinical Infectious Diseases 1994; 19:287-98.

104. Goodrich JM, Bowden RA, Fisher L, Keller C, Schoch G, Meyers JD. Ganciclovir prophylaxis to prevent cytomegalovirus disease after allogeneic marrow transplant. Annals of Internal Medicine 1993; 118:173-8.

105. Winston DJ, Ho WG, Bartoni K, Champlin RE. Intravenous immunoglobulin and CMV-seronegative blood products for prevention of CMV infection and disease in bone marrow transplant recipients. Bone Marrow Transplantation 1993; 12:283-8.

106. Guglielmo BJ, Wong-Beringer A, Linker CA. Immune globulin therapy in allogeneic bone marrow transplant: a critical review [see comments]. [Review] [21 refs]. Bone Marrow Transplantation 1994; 13:499-510.

107. Siadak MF, Kopecky K, Sullivan KM. Reduction in transplant-related complications in patients given intravenous immunoglobulin after allogeneic marrow transplantation. [Review] [55 refs]. Clinical & Experimental Immunology 1994; 97:53-7.

108. Atkinson K, Farwell V, Storb R et al. VZV infection after marrow transplantation for aplastic anemia or leukemia. Transplantation 1982; 29:47-50.

109. Caldas C, Ambinder R. Epstein-Barr virus and bone marrow transplantation [see comments]. [Review] [46 refs]. Current Opinion in Oncology 1995; 7:102-6.

110. Papadopoulos EB et al. Infusions of donor leukocytes to treat Epstein-Barr virus-associated lymphoproliferative disorders after allogeneic bone marrow transplantation [see comments]. New England Journal of Medicine 1994; 330:1185-91.

111. Russell N, Hunter A, Rogers S, Hanley J, Anderson D. Peripheral blood stem cells as an alternative to marrow for allogeneic transplantation. The Lancet 1993; 341:1482.

112. Dreger P, Suttorp M, Haferlack T, Loffler H, Schmitz N. Allogeneic granulocyte colony-stimulating factor-mobilized peripheral blood progenitor cells for treatment of engraftment failure after bone marrow transplantation. Blood 1993; 5:1404-1409.

113. Sasaki A et al. Transplantation of allogeneic peripheral blood stem cells after myeloablative treatment of a patient in a blastic crisis of chronic myelocytic leukemia. American Journal of Hematology 1994; 47:45-49.

114. To LB et al. Comparison of haematological recovery times and supportive care requirements of autologous recovery phase peripheral blood stem cell transplants, autologous bone marrow transplants and allogeneic bone marrow transplants. Bone Marrow Transplantation 1992; 9:277-84.

115. Buckner CD, Bensinger WI. Allogeneic peripheral blood stem cell transplantation. [Review] [23 refs]. Rinsho Ketsueki—Japanese Journal of Clinical Hematology 1997; 38:157-61.

116. Dreger P, Glass B, Uharek L, Schmitz N. Allogeneic peripheral blood progenitor cells: Current status and future directions. [Review] [65 refs]. Journal of Hematotherapy 1996; 5:331-7.

117. Aversa F et al. Successful engraftment of T cell-depleted haploident-ical "three loci" incompatible transplants in leukemia patients by addition of rhG-CSF-mobilized peripheral blood progenitor cells to bone marrow inoculum. 1994; 84:3948-3955.

118. Koc H et al. Is there an increased risk of graft-versus-host disease after allogeneic peripheral blood stem cell transplantation? [letter]. Blood 1996; 88:2362-4.

119. Davies SM, Ramsay NK, Haake RJ, Kersey JH, Weisdorf DJ, McGlave PB, Blazar BR. Comparison of engraftment in recipients of matched sibling of unrelated donor marrow allografts. Bone Marrow Transplantation 1994; 13:51-7.

120. Cullis JO et al. Matched unrelated donor bone marrow transplanta-tion for chronic myeloid leukaemia in chronic phase: comparison of ex vivo and in vivo T cell depletion. Bone Marrow Transplanta-tion 1993; 11:107-11.

121. Hensley-Downey P, Gee A, Godder K, Geler S. Minimal risk of graft versus host disease following haploidentical but partially mismatched related donor bone marrow transplantation. Exp Hem 1994; 22:716.

122. Nademanee A et al. The outcome of matched unrelated donor bone marrow transplantation in patients with hematologic malignancies using molecular typing for donor selection and graft-versus-host disease prophylaxis regimen of cyclosporine, methotrexate, and pred-nisone. Blood 1995; 86:1228-34.

123. Trigg ME. Bone marrow transplantation using alternative donors. Mismatched related donors or closely matched unrelated donors. [Review]. American Journal of Pediatric Hematology-Oncology 1993; 15:141-9.

124. Kernan N, Bartsch G, Ash R et al. Retrospective analysis of 462 un-related transplants facilitated by the National Marrow Donor Pro-gram for treatment of acquired and congenital disorders of the lymphohematopoietic system and congenital metabolic disorders. N Engl J Med 1993; 328:593-602.

125. Farrell C, Chapman J. Outcome of searches for a matched unrelated donor in the international registries. Transplantation Proceedings 1992; 24:179.

126. Martin P. Increased disparity for minor histocompatibility antigens as potential cause of increased GvHD risk in marrow transplanta-tion from unrelated donors compared with related donors. Bone Marrow Transplant 1991; 8:217-223.

127. Broxmeyer HE, Cooper S, Yoder M, Hangoc G. Human umbilical cord blood as a source of transplantable hematopoietic stem and progenitor cells. [Review]. Current Topics in Microbiology & Im-munology 1992; 177:195-204.

128. Wagner JE, Jr. Umbilical cord blood stem cell transplantation: cur-rent status and future prospects (1992). [Review]. Journal of Hematotherapy 1993; 2:225-8.

129. Kurtzberg J, Graham M, Casey J, Olson J, Stevens CE, Rubinstein P. The use of umbilical cord blood in mismatched related and unrelated hemopoietic stem cell transplantation. Blood Cells 1994; 20:275-83; discussion 284.

130. Gluckman E et al. Clinical applications of stem cell transfusion from cord blood and rationale for cord blood banking. [Review]. Bone Marrow Transplantation 1992; 9:114-7.

131. Cetrulo CL, Sbarra AJ, Cetrulo CL, Jr. Collection and cryopreservation of cord blood for the treatment of hematopoietic disorders: the obstetrician's overview. Journal of Hematotherapy 1996; 5:149-51.

132. Rubinstein P et al. Processing and cryopreservation of placental/ umbilical cord blood for unrelated bone marrow reconstitution. Proc Natl Acad Sci USA 1995; 92:10119-22.

133. Campos L, Roubi N, Guyotat D. Definition of optimal conditions for collection and cryopreservation of umbilical cord hematopoietic cells. Cryobiology 1995; 32:511-5.

134. Bertolini F, Lazzari L, Corsini C, Lauri E, Gorini F, Sirchia G. Cord blood banking for stem cell transplant. International Journal of Artificial Organs 1993; 16:111-2.

135. Dracker RA. Cord blood stem cells: how to get them and what to do with them. Journal of Hematotherapy 1996; 5:145-8.

136. Gluckman E, Wagner J, Hows J, Kernan N, Bradley B, Broxmeyer HE. Cord blood banking for hematopoietic stem cell transplantation: an international cord blood transplant registry. Bone Marrow Transplantation 1993; 11:199-200.

137. Wagner J, Kernan N, Steinbuch M, Broxmeyer H, Gluckman E. Allogeneic sibling umbilical cord blood transplantation in children with malignant and nonmalignant disease. Lancet 1995; 346: 214-219.

138. Kurtzberg J et al. Single center transplantation of HLA matched partially mismatched unrelated placental blood: An alternative source od hematopoietic stem cells for bone marrow transplantation. New England J of Med 1996; 335:157-166.

139. Rubinstein P et al. Unrelated placental blood for bone marrow reconstitution: organization of the placental blood program [see comments]. Blood Cells 1994; 20:587-96; discussion 596-600.

140. Rubinstein P et al. New York Blood Center's program for unrelated placental/umbilical cord blood transplantation: 243 transplants in the first 3 years. Blood 1996; 10 (sup 1):142a.

141. Kurtzberg J, Laughlin M, Smith C et al. Hematopoietic recovery in adult recipients following unrelated umbilical cord blood transplantation. Blood 1997; 90 (supp 1):110a.

142. Kogler G et al. Hematopoietic transplant potential of unrelated cord blood: Critical issues. Journal of Hematotherapy 1996; 5:105-16.

143. Broxmeyer HE et al. Growth characteristics and expansion of human umbilical cord blood and estimation of its potential for transplantation in adults. Proceedings of the National Academy of Sciences of the United States of America 1992; 89:4109-13.

144. DiGiusto DL et al. Hematopoietic potential of cryopreserved and ex vivo manipulated umbilical cord blood progenitor cells evaluated in vitro and in vivo. Blood 1996; 87:1261-1271.

145. Van Zant G, Rummel SA, Koller MR, Larson DB, Drubachevsky I, Palsson M, Emerson SG. Expansion in bioreactors of human progenitor populations from cord blood and mobilized peripheral blood [see comments]. Blood Cells 1994; 20:482-90; discussion 491.

146. Kohn DB. The current status of gene therapy using hematopoietic stem cells. [Review]. Curr Opin Pediatr 1995; 7:56-63.

147. Moritz T, Keller DC, Williams DA. Human cord blood cells as targets for gene transfer: Potential use in genetic therapies of severe combined immunodeficiency disease. Journal of Experimental Medicine 1993; 178:529-36.

148. Williams DA, Moritz T. Umbilical cord blood stem cells as targets for genetic modification: new therapeutic approaches to somatic gene therapy. Blood Cells 1994; 20:504-15; discussion 515-6.

149. Gill Pet al.. AIDS-related malignant lymphoma: Results of prospective treatment trials. Journal of Clinical Oncology 1987; 5:1322-1328.

150. Gisselbrecht C et al. Human immunodeficiency virus-related lymphoma treatment with intensive combination chemotherapy. French-Italian Cooperative Group. American Journal of Medicine 1993; 95:188-96.

151. Levine A. Acquired immunodeficiency syndrome-related lymphoma. Blood 1992; 80:8-20.

152. Contu L et al. Allogeneic bone marrow transplantation combined with multiple anti-HIV-1 treatment in a case of AIDS. Bone Marrow Transplantation 1993; 12:669-671.

153. Williams DA. Syngeneic bone marrow transplantation and failure to eradicate HIV. AIDS 1991; 5:344.

154. Torlontano G et al. AIDS-related complex treated by antiviral drugs and allogeneic bone marrow transplantation following conditioning protocol with busulphan, cyclophosphamide and cyclosporin. Haematologica 1992; 77:287-90.

155. Cooper M, Maraninchi D, Gastaut J, Mannoni P, Caracassonne Y. HIV infection in autologous and allogeneic bone marrow transplant patients: a retrospective analysis of the Marseille bone marrow transplant population. Journal of Acquired Immune Deficiency Syndrome 1993; 6:277-284.

156. Holland H et al. Allogeneic bone marrow transplantation, zidovudine, and human immunodeficiency virus type 1 (HIV-1) infection. Annals of Internal Medicine 1989; 111:973-981.

157. Mellonig JT, Prewett AB, Moyer MP. HIV inactivation in a bone allograft. J Periodontol 1992; 63:979-83.

158. Bandini G, Re M, Rosti G, Beardinelli A. HIV infection and bone-marrow transplantation. The Lancet 1991; 337:1163-1164.

159. Angelucci E, Lucarelli G, Baronciani D, Durazzi SM, Galimberti M, Maddaloni D, Polchi P. Bone marrow transplantation in an HIV positive thalassemic child following therapy with azidothymidine. Haematologica 1990; 75:285-7.

160. Jootar S, Angchaisuksiri P, Chiewsilp P, Sathapatayavongs B, Chuncharunee S, Tanprasert S. HIV infection after autologous bone marrow transplantation despite HIV-antibody and HIV-antigen screening. Bone Marrow Transplantation 1993; 12:167-8.

161. Turner M, Watson H, Russell L, Langlands K, Parker A, Parker, CA. An HIV positive haemophiliac with acute lymphoblastic leukaemia successfully treated with intensive chemotherapy syngeneic bone marrow transplantation. Bone Marrow Transplantation 1992; 9:387-389.

162. Saral R, Holland H. Bone Marrow Transplantation for the Acquired Immune Deficiency Syndrome. In: Forman S, Blume K, Thomas E, eds. Bone Marrow Transplantation. Boston: Blackwell Scientific Publishers 1994.

163. Klinman DM, Krieg A, Conover J, Ussery MA, Black PL. Effect of cyclophosphamide, total body irradiation, and zidovudine on retrovirus proliferation and disease progression in murine AIDS. Aids Research & Human Retroviruses 1992; 8:101-6.

164. Fultz P. Total lymphoid irradiation as a novel therapeutic approach for treatment of HIV-induced disease. 1993.

165. Levine AM et al. Human immunodeficiency virus-related lymphoma. Prognostic factors predictive of survival. Cancer 1991; 68:2466-72.

166. Caliendo AM, Hirsch MS. Combination therapy for infection due to human immunodeficiency virus type 1 [published erratum appears in Clin Infect Dis 1994 Aug;19(2):379]. [Review]. Clinical Infectious Diseases 1994; 18:516-24.

167. Deeks SG, Smith M, Holodniy M, Kahn JO. HIV-1 protease inhibitors. A review for clinicians. [Review] [59 refs]. Jama 1997; 277:145-53.

168. McDonald CK, Kuritzkes DR. Human immunodeficiency virus type 1 protease inhibitors. [Review] [86 refs]. Archives of Internal Medicine 1997; 157:951-9.

169. Takada A, Takada Y, Ambrus J. Proliferation of donor spleen and bone marrow cells in the spleen and bone marrow of unirradiated and irradiated adult mice. Proc Soc Exp Biol Med 1970; 136:222.

170. Micklem J et al. Fate of chromosome marked mouse bone marrow cells transfused into normal syngeneic recipients. Transplantation 1968; 6:299.

171. Ramshaw HS, Crittenden RB, Dooner M, Peters SO, Rao SS, Quesenberry PJ. High levels of engraftment with a single infusion of bone marrow cells into normal unprepared mice [published erratum appears in Biol Blood Marrow Transplant 1996 Feb;2(1):54]. Biology of Blood and Marrow Transplantation 1995; 1:74-80.

172. Quesenberry PJ et al. Engraftment of normal murine marrow into nonmyeloablated host mice. Blood Cells 1994; 20:348-50.

173. Ramshaw HS, Rao SS, Crittenden RB, Peters SO, Weier HU, Quesenberry PJ. Engraftment of bone marrow cells into normal unprepared hosts: effects of 5-fluorouracil and cell cycle status. Blood 1995; 86:924-9.

174. Rao SS, Peters SO, Crittenden RB, Stewart FM, Ramshaw HS, Quesenberry PJ. Stem cell transplantation in the normal non-myeloablated host: relationship between cell dose, schedule, and engraftment. Experimental Hematology 1997; 25:114-21.

175. Stewart F, Crittenden R, Lowry P, Pearson-White S, Quesenberry P. Long-term engraftment of normal and post-5-fluorouracil murine marrow into nonmyeloablated mice. Blood 1993; 81:2566-2571.

176. Nilsson SK, Dooner MS, Tiarks CY, Weier HU, Quesenberry PJ. Potential and distribution of transplanted hematopoietic stem cells in a nonablated mouse model. Blood 1997; 89:4013-20.

177. Mardiney MR, Malech HL. Enhanced engraftment of hematopoietic progenitor cells in mice treated with granulocyte colony-stimulating factor before low-dose irradiation: Implications for gene therapy. Blood 1996; 87:4049-56.

178. Mardiney MR, Jackson SH, Spratt SK, Li F, Holland SM, Malech HL. Enhanced host defense after gene transfer in the murine p47phox-deficient model of chronic granulomatous disease. Blood 1997; 89:2268-75.

179. Khouri I, Przepiorka D, van Besien K et al. Allogeneic blood or marrow transplantation for chronic lymphocytic leukaemia: timing of transplantation and potential effect of fludarabine on acute graft-versus-host disease. British Journal of Haematology 1997; 97:466-73.

180. Baum C, Hegewisch-Becker S, Eckert HG, Stocking C, Ostertag W. Novel retroviral vectors for efficient expression of the multidrug resistance (mdr-1) gene in early hematopoietic cells. Journal of Virology 1995; 69:7541-7.

181. Hanania EG, Fu S, Roninson I, Zu Z, Gottesman MM, Deisseroth AB. Resistance to taxol chemotherapy produced in mouse marrow cells by safety-modified retroviruses containing a human MDR-1 transcription unit [see comments]. Gene Ther 1995; 2:279-84.

182. Richardson C, Ward M, Bank A. MDR gene transfer into live mice. [Review] [51 refs]. Journal of Molecular Medicine 1995; 73:189-95.

183. Hanania EG et al. Results of MDR-1 vector modification trial indicate that granulocyte/macrophage colony-forming unit cells do not contribute to posttransplant hematopoietic recovery following intensive systemic therapy [published erratum appears in Proc Natl Acad Sci USA 1997 May 13;94(10):5495]. Proceedings of the National Academy of Sciences of the United States of America 1996; 93:15346-51.

184. Hesdorffer C, Antman K, Bank A, Fetell M, Mears G, Begg M. Human MDR gene transfer in patients with advanced cancer. Human Gene Therapy 1994; 5:1151-60.

185. Cavert W, Notermans D, Staskus K et al. Kinetics of response in lymphoid tissues to antiretroviral therapy of HIV-1 infection. Science 276:960-964.

186. Dunbar CE, Emmons RV. Gene transfer into hematopoietic progenitor and stem cells: Progress and problems. [Review]. Stem Cells (Dayt) 1994; 12:563-76.

187. Bordignon C, Mavillo F, Ferrari G. Transfer of the ADA gene into bone marrow cells and peripheral blood lymphocytes for the treatment of patients affected by ADA deficient SCID. Human Gene Therapy 1993; 4:513.

Index